Fit & Healthy Forever

Fit & Healthy Forever

✦

Joe Barrett

iUniverse, Inc.
New York Bloomington

Fit & Healthy Forever

You should not undertake any diet/exercise regimen recommended in this book before consulting your personal physician. Neither the author nor the publisher shall be responsible or liable for any loss or damage allegedly arising as a consequence of your use or application of any information or suggestions contained in this book.

iUniverse books may be ordered through booksellers or by contacting:

iUniverse
1663 Liberty Drive
Bloomington, IN 47403
www.iuniverse.com
1-800-Authors (1-800-288-4677)

Because of the dynamic nature of the Internet, any Web addresses or links contained in this book may have changed since publication and may no longer be valid. The views expressed in this work are solely those of the author and do not necessarily reflect the views of the publisher, and the publisher hereby disclaims any responsibility for them.

ISBN:978-0-595-44354-3 (pbk)
ISBN:978-0-595-88683-8 (ebk)
ISBN:978-0-595-70039-4 cloth)

Printed in the United States of America

Front cover photograph Mitsuru Okabe
The back cover and inside flap photograph JM Manion

IUniverse revision date: 6/5/2009

In memory of John J. Barrett, 1958–2000

Contents

8. Basic Weight-Training Exercises 57

9. Cardiovascular Exercise (Aerobic Conditioning)....119

10. Workout Schedules and Routines 125

Acknowledgments

I would like to thank everyone who has helped make this book possible. Some have motivated and inspired me. Others have acted as role models and mentors who helped point me in the right direction.

Most of all, I would like to thank God for giving me this wonderful life. I would also like to thank my mother and father for giving me their unconditional love and support, for always believing in me, and for being there for me through the good times and the bad. I feel blessed to have had the opportunity to share my love, friendship and many wonderful experiences with my brother John. I would like to express my deepest gratitude to Jim Parsells, who has played a very special part in my life and always knew how to get me motivated. I would like to express my love and appreciation to Kathy Marino, Savannah, and Cody, for bringing love and happiness into my life. I am grateful to have Sunny Barrett as part of my family and I appreciate all of her love and kindness.

A special thanks to MuscleTech Research And Development (www. muscletech.com) for believing in me and turning my dreams into reality, especially for introducing me to their cutting-edge supplements that helped transform my physique into what it is today. My good friend, training partner, and fellow competitor John Wood has been my mentor and has served as a role model for me in the sport of bodybuilding. Sincere thanks to Terry Giovinazzo for her neverending unconditional friendship, her priceless help, and for always making me feel like a winner. I am privileged to have as a friend Cyndi James, a pro bodybuilder who has always given me advice and professional guidance: she has shown me by example that with hard work and dedication you can succeed. I express my gratitude to Terry Goodlad for his friendship as well as his excellent photography and writing skills, and most of all for opening doors to many opportunities and truly making me feel like a superstar. I am extremely grateful for my friendship with bodybuilding and fitness extraordinaire Dr. Alfred K. Thomas, His positive attitude and wealth of knowledge are second to none. The world is a better place because he is in it. I would like to express deep appreciation to my good friend and training partner Bob Powers for, many years of his friendship and support. I am blessed to have as a friend Bill Blake, a motivated training partner, and an excellent role model. Thanks to Dr. Arthur G. Nahas, for his friendship and for keeping me healthy. I would like to convey my gratitude to Ken Haring for his years of unconditional friendship and support. This book would probably still be just an idea without my friend and fellow author, George Pappadopoulos, pushing me to write it. I would also like to acknowledge some additional friends who have had a positive impact on my life. Rob Rambo, Tod Settle, Robbie Reilly, Steve Weeks, Dr. Lou Demoulin, John Varallo, Dr. Larry D. Lemieux, and Gary Jernee.

I would also like to recognize and thank particular individual athletes who have motivated and inspired me: Arnold Schwarzenegger, Steve Reeves, Mike Antorino, Bruce Lee, Kurt Thomas, Mary Lou Retton, Florence Griffith-Jointer, Lou Ferrigno, Jack Lalanne, Rich Gaspari, Francis Benfatto, Bob Paris, Roland Kikinger, Dexter Jackson, Frank Zepe, Flex Wheeler, Stan McQuay, Mike Matarazzo, Bill Pearl, Robbie Robinson, Mike Matarazzo, Tom Platz, Milos Sarcev, Lee Haney, Lee Labrada, Franco Columbo, Kevin Lavrone, Denise Rutkawski, Tony Pearson, Vince Taylor, Gunter Schlierkamp, and Ronnie Coleman. In addition, special thanks to Somers Point Gymnastic Center, Vineland Gymnastic Center, Atlantic Gymnastics Academy, Cape Gymnastic World Inc., Glassboro State Gymnastics, Gold's Gym, Somers Point Fitness, Muscle World Gym, The Spa At Bally's and Ateamxtreme (www.ateamxtreme.com).

The author at a photo shoot for Muscle East Video

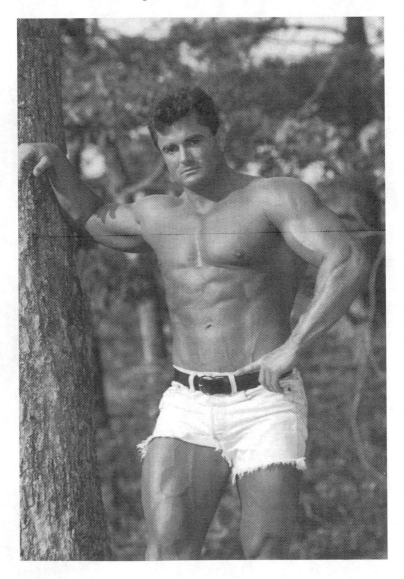

Photo by Muscle East Video

Author's Note

I have devoted my life to health and fitness. After competing in collegiate gymnastics as team captain, I focused on bodybuilding. As a competitive bodybuilder I earned the title of Mr. Garden State and received trophies in many other prestigious contests, including Mr. USA and Mr. America. These accomplishments ultimately landed me a spot performing with the Chippendale dance revue. In addition, I have appeared in dozens of fitness magazines and on national television promoting health and fitness.

One of my greatest accomplishments was my first place finish in one of the largest contests in the history of bodybuilding. Over forty thousand contestants entered and my grand prize included more than $100,000 in cash and prizes. Winning this contest is one of the reasons I was inspired to write this book and share my vast knowledge of the health and fitness field. My hope is that this book will help others to succeed as I have and reach their dreams.

Education

Associate in Science Degree

Licensed Massage Therapist – New Jersey Board of Nursing (Licensed/Certified/Registered)

Certified Personal Trainer – American Aerobics Association International - AAAI & International Sports Medicine Association - ISMA

Athletic Accomplishments

1982–83 Captain Glassboro State College Gymnastics Team

1986 A.A.U. Atlantic Coast Bodybuilding Championships—2nd Place Light Weight

1986 A.A.U. Garden State Bodybuilding Championships—1st Place Light Weight

1987 N.P.C New Jersey Classic Bodybuilding Championships-3rd Place Light Weight

1989 A.A.U. USA. Bodybuilding Championships—5th Place Medium Class

1995 N.P.C. Muscle Beach Bodybuilding Championships—2nd Place Middle Weight

1995 N.P.C. Muscle Beach Bodybuilding Championships—2nd Place Masters

1995 A.A.U. Mr. America Bodybuilding Championships—4th Place Light Weight

1996 N.P.C. Collegiate National Bodybuilding Championships—3rd Place Middle Weight

2000 N.P.C. Jan Tana Classic Bodybuilding Championships—3rd Place Middle Weight

2000 N.P.C. Jan Tana Classic Bodybuilding Championships— 2nd Place Masters

2000 MuscleTech Millennium Physique Transformation Contest—1st Place Men Over Thirty

2000 MuscleTech Millennium Physique Transformation Contest—1st Place Grand Champion

2000 Galaxy Regional Fitness Competition—Top Finisher

2002 N.P.C. Masters National Bodybuilding Championships—8th Place Middle Weight

2002 N.P.C Jan Tana Classic Bodybuilding Championships-2nd Place Middle Weight

Other Accomplishments

1987 Performed in the Chippendale Dance Revue

2000 *Baywatch* TV show talent search contest—Top Five Male Finisher

Magazines Appearances

- MuscleMag International
- Oxygen
- American Health & Fitness
- Bodysport
- Muscle & Fitness
- Muscle & Fitness Hers
- Flex
- Men's Fitness
- Men's Exercise
- Men's Workout
- Exercise for Men Only
- Muscle Media
- Muscular Development
- Ironman
- Irony
- Bodytalk
- Physical
- Let's Live
- Great Life
- Mind & Muscle Power
- NPC News
- Natural Muscle Magazine
- Natural Bodybuilding & Fitness
- Casino Journal
- Viper Magazine
- Fun 'N' Games
- Playgirl

Preface

Perhaps because I have always kept in very good physical condition, I probably look like a walking advertisement for health and fitness. For many years I have been approached almost daily and bombarded with questions concerning proper diet and exercise. At first I tried to communicate the necessary information verbally, but that became very tedious. Therefore, I started writing it down and handing it out to friends, coworkers, gym members, etc. After several years of distributing these written materials, I ultimately decided to put all of my knowledge into book form.

The focus of this book is to educate you about the numerous variables that contribute to constructing and maintaining a successful exercise and diet program. Keep in mind, there is no one factor that will create your success. A combination of factors will determine how much progress you make, and how quickly you obtain it. I repeatedly hear the same question: *"How long will it take me to get into shape?"* Because many variables will play a role in the progress of your workouts, it is difficult to predict a specific outcome. The following is a partial list of factors that can affect the speed of your progress.

- Consistency

- Intensity

- Proper diet

- Sleep

- Nutritional supplements

- Age

- Genetics

- Metabolism

- Gender

- Weight

- Lifestyle

The author at a photo shoot for *Bodysport Magazine*

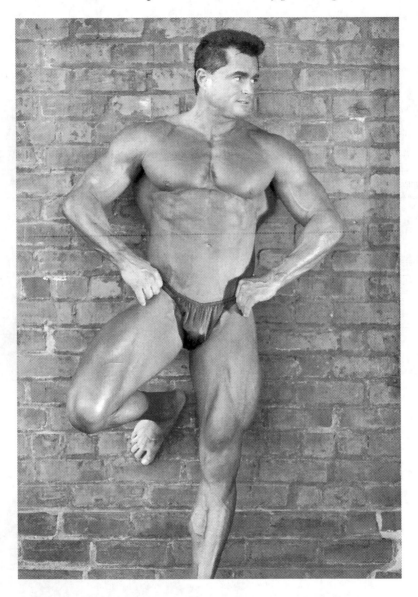

Photo by Terry Goodlad (www.bodysport.com)

Introduction

How I got in the best shape of my life and won over $100,000 for doing it

Knowing about diet and exercise is only one part of a fitness program. Following through with what you have learned is the only way you will achieve actual results. I had more than enough knowledge about diet and exercise, but one day I realized that I was not putting it to work for me. The bottom line: I was not practicing what I preached. But all that changed; let me share my personal success story with you.

It all began when I hit the big "four-zero." It seemed to mark a time for self-assessment and soul-searching. All it took was one look in the mirror! I had always been a good athlete, in excellent physical condition, but now I had somehow slipped off the path. Growing up I participated in many sports, ultimately excelling in gymnastics. After college I entered several bodybuilding contests and always placed very high. However, over time, my workouts slowly began to diminish. I did work out, but I did not apply the intensity or the consistency I once had. And my diet had fallen by the wayside.

I was normally disciplined in my workouts and diet, yet I knew I was in a rut. I needed a goal to get back into shape. While reading a fitness magazine one day, I came across an ad for a "Physique Transformation Contest" sponsored by MuscleTech, a nutritional supplement company. "All you have to do is get in the best shape of your life," stated the ad. The contest included several different categories: Beginners, Advanced, Women's Open, Men 18 to 29, Men over 30, and Fat Loss. "Bingo!" I said. "This is just what I need!"

The contest consisted of writing an eight-hundred-word essay, completing a several-page booklet with questions, statistics et cetera, and submitting before-and-after photographs. The essay addressed the following questions.

- Why did you get involved in weight training?

- What are your long-term goals?

- How has getting in shape affected your life?

- What type of weight training did you follow?

- What type of diet did you follow and for how long?

- What supplements (if any) did you select to transform your physique and how have they helped you?

The photos consisted of predetermined poses in front, side, and back views. The before photos had to be taken prior to starting your diet and exercise program. The after pictures were to be taken approximately twelve weeks later. I decided to enter the "Men over 30" category and immediately began to establish my goals. I needed to completely reconstruct my workout and diet, and I wanted to add some new high-tech supplements to the program.

I scheduled additional workout days and incorporated a double-split routine (work out twice a day: once in the morning and once in the evening). I focused on training my weaker body parts (priority training), and added a substantial amount of cardiovascular exercise.

At the start, my diet was sloppy and my physique reflected it. I immediately changed from three to four large meals per day to six to eight smaller meals. I also limited my fat, sodium, and sugar intake. My meals consisted of chicken, fish, and egg whites for protein and rice, potatoes, and fresh vegetables for carbohydrates.

Next came the "icing on the cake": nutritional supplements. I have always believed that you get what you pay for, so instead of wasting my money on no-name bogus brands, I chose a well-established company that funds research and development at several universities to continuously improve its products. I was confident that its products were safe and effective.

I chose a thermogentic (a fat burner), a protein powder (for high-quality protein), and a meal replacement (shakes/bars). After approximately twelve weeks had passed, I was ready to take my after photographs and record my new statistics. I had lost twenty-two pounds of fat (from 19.6 percent body fat down to 4.3 percent), and reduced my waistline by six inches. I had also increased my bench press by fifty pounds.

Several months passed after I entered the contest. Then one day I received a phone call from the nutritional supplement company that had sponsored it: I was one of the top ten winners. The representative told me I had won over $32,000 in cash and prizes and was in the running for the grand prize, a Dodge Viper sports car valued at over $72,000.

Several days later, the rep called again and asked me, "Joe, do you have a garage?" I told him I did and he said, "You're the grand prize winner!" As part of my prize package, I was flown to the Arnold Schwarzenegger Classic Bodybuilding and Fitness Show, where I was scheduled for some professional photo shoots. During my visit I had the opportunity to meet several bodybuilding stars such as Arnold Schwarzenegger and Lou Ferrigno ("The Incredible Hulk"). I also met many other prominent individuals in the sport.

As a result of winning that first contest I've been featured in dozens of magazines, and have received network news coverage. Above and beyond the original prize package, the nutritional supplement company asked me if I would be interested in participating in its first national TV commercial. Of course I was eager to accept another once-in-a-lifetime opportunity.

I believe that no matter what the outcome of the contest might have been, I was already a winner. The entire experience not only improved my physique and energy level, but also enhanced my self-esteem and self-confidence.

I hope that I can serve as a role model for anyone at any age. I believe that anyone can achieve whatever they want in life if they have the will. Always maintain a positive attitude and stay focused. If you do, I believe that there is absolutely nothing you cannot accomplish.

The author's before-and-after pictures

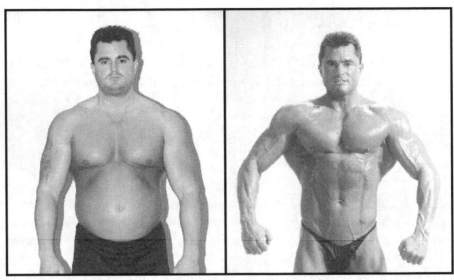

Before   After

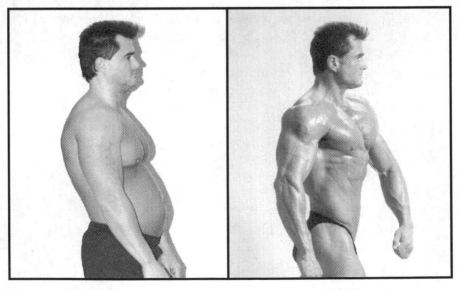

Before   After

The author with Arnold Schwarzenegger

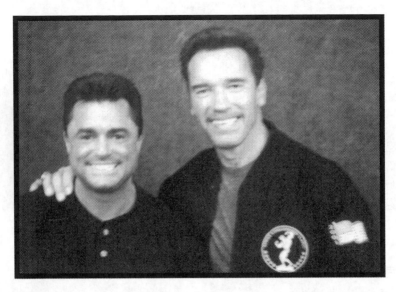

The author with Lou Ferrigno
("The Incredible Hulk")

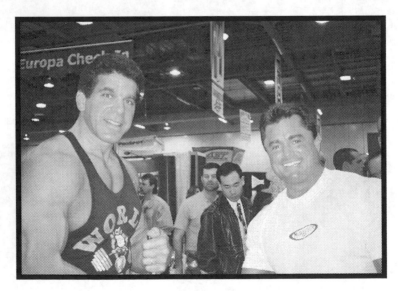

1

Understanding Your Body

Benefits of Exercise

Exercise can enhance the overall quality of your life physically, mentally, and spiritually. The following is a small list illustrating some benefits of exercise.

- Control weight, prevent obesity

- Help reduce LDL (bad) cholesterol levels

- Help reduce blood sugar levels

- Slow the aging process

- Increase your energy level

- Help improve sleep

- Help prevent heart disease

- Help rehabilitate after injury, operation, or illness

- Help fight depression

- Reduce anxiety

- Help relieve stress

- Increase self-esteem

- Increase self-confidence

Genetics

Genetics involves the genes you inherit from your parents before birth. While they will determine things such as your height, weight, symmetry, and the basic size and shape of your muscles, exercising can tone and reshape your muscles. Genetics can also dictate the rate of your metabolism and the amount of body fat you normally possess, although diet and exercise can manipulate these factors as well.

As you experiment with your exercise program, you will discover how quickly you as an individual respond to diet and exercise. You may come to find that one area of your body carries more fat than another. You may also discover that you have one or two exceptional body parts that will respond faster to exercise than others.

Remember, your genetic makeup was determined before you were born. Therefore, some individuals will have to diet and exercise harder than others to achieve similar results as someone with superior genetics.

Metabolism

Metabolism converts the food we eat into fuel to supply the body with energy for physical movement, thinking, and growing. Each person's metabolism is unique; some people can eat all day and not gain a pound and others watch their intake carefully and cannot lose a pound. Many factors play a role in determining a specific individual's metabolism: age, genetics, gender, weight, and "body composition" (amount of muscle and fat). A person who has more lean muscle and less fat on his frame will burn more calories at rest than a person who is overweight or obese.

- **Anabolism** is *constructive metabolism*: It supports the growth of new cells, helps maintain body tissues, and stores energy for future use.

- **Catabolism** is *destructive metabolism*: Catabolism breaks down large molecules to release energy for the body.

- **Resting metabolic rate (RMR) or basal metabolic rate (BMR)** is the number of calories that an individual will burn in a state of rest. RMR or BMR reflects the caloric need to maintain basic physiological functions, breathing, circulating blood, and organ function.

Misconceptions

There are several misconceptions concerning the physiological effects of weight training and I would like to clear up a few of them.

The Age Factor

Workouts can be conducted at any age; however, the intensity may vary with the individual. As a general rule, the aging process will slow down your resting metabolic rate (RMR); therefore, as your metabolism becomes slower you burn fewer calories. As you age your potential to tone or build muscle will probably be negatively affected as well. Also recuperating from your workouts may take a bit longer.

In addition, our joints possess only a certain amount of mileage, per individual, per lifetime. Wear and tear on joints over the years may ultimately restrict your physical capabilities. Joints are mostly made up of ligaments, tendons, and cartilage. When injured, these tissues usually take quite a bit of time to heal and regenerate. Muscle tissue is more vascular (rich in blood) than joint-related tissues; therefore, muscles regenerate and heal much more rapidly. Enhancing your muscles with a workout program can help to support weak joints.

In sum, the only issue to consider regarding age is that you may have to work harder and smarter to achieve similar results to a younger person's. Nevertheless, do not let age be a factor when considering whether to work out or not!

Fat and Muscle

There is a common myth I have heard many times: *"When you stop working out, all your muscles turn to fat."* This transformation is absolutely impossible; one type of body tissue cannot turn into another. What actually happens involves two processes. First, when you stop exercising, muscles will atrophy (become smaller). Second, you will probably accumulate more body fat (providing you maintain the same diet). This creates the illusion that the muscles have turned to fat. To sum it all up, if you stop exercising you will more than likely end up in the same shape you were in prior to exercising.

As I mentioned earlier in the metabolism section, your total body weight or body composition (amount of muscle and fat) is very important in keeping body fat to a minimum. People who possess more lean muscle and less fat on their frames will burn more calories even while sitting or sleeping than those who are overweight or obese.

As you progress with your diet and exercise program, you will lose body fat and gain muscle. Muscle cells are a denser tissue than fat cells; fat takes up approximately five times the space of muscle. Your actual weight may not change too dramatically, but you should become smaller in size. I will discuss this more in chapter 3 ("Body Fat").

Women and Muscle

Many women repeat this cliché: "Weight training will give me bulky, manly muscle." But women need not be concerned with getting bulky; it will not happen by accident. It would require many years of extremely intense hard-core bodybuilding to achieve that level of muscle. Such an attitude is like saying "I had better not take piano lessons, because I will not be able to afford the dress I will want to wear when I play at Carnegie Hall." Let us be realistic; you simply will not inadvertently get bulky muscles from weight training. Using weight training, women can tone and shape their bodies without building bulky muscle. Consider your body as a piece of clay; weight training can help you reshape and transform it into a shape that you desire.

The author at a photo shoot for MuscleTech

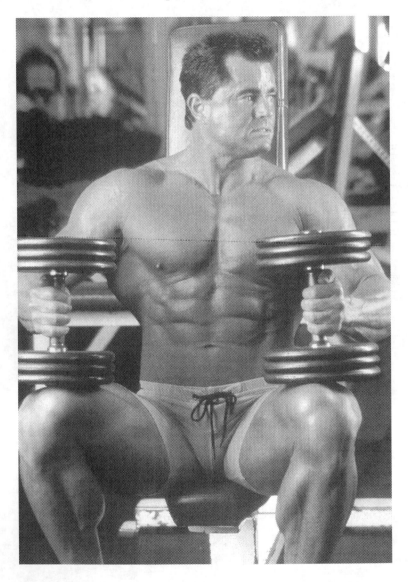

Photo by Mitsuru Okabe (www.mocvideo.com)

2

Getting Started

How to Get Motivated

It is time to get motivated! You must ask yourself, "What are the main reasons for starting an exercise program?" You may have multiple reasons. Try to visualize your reasons for wanting to improve your physical condition, before and during your workouts. Mental imagery is a powerful tool.

Personally, I like to use photographs of individuals who motivate me—they could be male or female. Clip out pictures that appeal to you from magazines and use them as role models. Choose pictures that that will give you the desire to improve your physical appearance. Look at them on the days when you feel like skipping a workout or when you need to get extra motivated for a tough workout after a hard day.

Perhaps you are overweight or obese and therefore have low self-confidence, low self-esteem, low energy level, or possibly even depression. The desire to lose weight to feel better about yourself can certainly be a good motivational tool. Maybe you would like to improve your physical appearance before attending a reunion or other special event. You may feel that you have become physically undesirable to your significant other and you want to look better to get his or her attention; never take for granted that your partner will always desire your physical appearance. I have seen people achieve remarkable results, rebounding from rejection following a failed relationship or marriage. Rehabilitation following a physical illness or injury is also a great motivator.

Exercising can help fight the mood swings, anxiety, and depression that occur for some women during menstruation. During pregnancy, a woman's body goes through a complete metamorphosis; wanting to get back to your original physical condition can help to motivate you to exercise. An exercise program can help manage and reduce many of the undesirable symptoms related to menopause and andropause (male menopause). Listed below are some more detailed examples of how exercise can help you with rehabilitation, pregnancy, menopause, and andropause.

Rehabilitation and Exercise

Injuries, operations, and illnesses usually leave the body impaired. Exercising can help support and heal weakened areas of your body after a physical setback.

Lower back pain is common in today's society: sciatica, herniated disk, fractured vertebra, et cetera. Sit-ups and lower back exercises can help strengthen and support your torso, helping to relieve lower back pain.

Knee injuries seem to be another common problem with many people. Exercising the quadriceps of the leg muscles can help *give additional support* to your knees and pick up the slack of a weak joint.

Internal surgeries such as, cancer operations, organ removal, and C-sections, involve cutting through muscle and other healthy tissues. Countless exercises can help rehabilitate the affected muscles.

Stroke victims often develop partial paralysis. Physical therapy involving a light exercise program is beneficial to recovery and rehabilitation.

Broken bones normally are put into a cast for an extended period of time. As a result, the immobilization of the area will cause the muscle to atrophy (become smaller). Physical therapy in the form of proper weight training is often required to help rebuild the lost muscle tissue.

Heart attacks affect a large percentage of today's population. Soon after a heart attack and/or heart surgery, most physicians recommend that a patient incorporate an exercise program into his or her lifestyle. Quite often, the core of the program is cardiovascular exercise to help strengthen the heart muscle, causing the heart to pump blood more efficiently. This in turn will help to keep the individual's body fat at a lower rate while building healthier arteries.

Automobile accidents are very prevalent in our world; almost everyone has been involved in one or knows someone who has. Those who undergo auto accidents are generally left with injuries that require some form of rehabilitation. In almost every case, physical therapy involving a weight-training program is initiated to help expedite recovery and get the victim as close to normal as possible.

These are only a few examples of how exercise aids in rehabilitation; each person will have his or her own particular circumstances.

Pregnancy and Exercise

Before exercising during pregnancy, you should consult your physician, physiotherapist, or other health care professional. This will help prevent harm to both you and your unborn baby. Below is a list of some of the benefits to be derived from exercise during pregnancy.

During pregnancy, a woman's body goes through major changes. This transformation takes an immense toll on the entire body. After giving birth, most new mothers are left with excess body fat, nonexistent muscle tone, and sometimes even lower back pain. A combination of muscular conditioning, aerobic exercise, and stretching can be beneficial before, during (under the guidance of a physician), and after pregnancy. In addition, post-pregnancy is a perfect time to establish an exercise program to help speed up the recovery process. The following are some benefits acquired from exercising during and after pregnancy.

- Look better

- Feel better

- Relieve stress

- Help fight fatigue

- Increase stamina

- Help balance hormones

- Help lessen morning sickness

- Strengthen back muscles

- Improve posture

- Gain less body fat

- Prepare for the physical demands of labor

- Speed up recuperation after labor

- Expedite the return to normal body weight

- Help prepare for the physical demands of motherhood

Before you begin exercising, make sure that you take the time to warm up thoroughly. Keep your exercise to moderate levels of intensity. Exercise on soft surfaces and wear a support bra if necessary. Drink plenty of water before, during, and after exercising. The following are some of the physical activities and exercises you may want to include during pregnancy.

- Walking

- Swimming

- Cycling (stationary bicycle)

- Stretching

- Yoga

- Dancing

- Exercise in water (aqua aerobics)

- Low-impact aerobics

- Pregnancy exercise classes

- Weight training (light weights, medium to high repetitions)

Below is a list of some physical activity and exercises to avoid during pregnancy.

- Sit-ups and crunches

- Outdoor cycling

- Rollerblading, roller-skating, ice-skating

- Contact sports

- Competitive sports

- Trampoline

- High-impact aerobics

If you experience any of the following, stop exercising immediately and contact your doctor.

- Dizziness

- Headache

- Difficulty walking

- Intense back pain

- Contractions

- Chest pain

- Heart palpitations

- Swelling of the face, hands, or feet

- Pain or swelling of calves

- Cramping of the lower abdomen

- Vaginal bleeding

- Amniotic fluid leakage

Let your instinct guide you. If you do not feel like exercising, do not push yourself; instead, rest and reserve your energy.

Menopause and Exercise

Premenopause, perimenopause, menopause (final menstrual cycle), and **postmenopause** can create drastic fluctuations in hormone levels such as estrogen, progesterone, and testosterone. Many negative side effects, both physiological and psychological, can be associated with these changes.

From premenopause through postmenopause, symptoms may last up to twenty years. Most women can expect all stages of menopause to last between four and five years, Women may experience changes in hormones as early as their thirties and up to their sixties. However, the average age of menopause occurs at around fifty-one years of age.

An exercise program including weight training, aerobic exercise, and stretching can help manage and reduce many of the undesirable symptoms related to the various phases involved with menopause. The following list contains some of the benefits of regular exercise in reducing the negative side effects.

- Reduce risk of heart disease

- Reduce risk of weight gain

- Reduce risk of osteoporosis

- Reduce fatigue

- Reduce headaches

- Reduce hot flashes

- Reduce joint pain

- Reduce anxiety

- Reduce depression

- Reduce irritability

- Reduce sleep disorders (insomnia)

Additional methods such as diet, nutritional supplements, and hormone replacement therapy (HRT) can also help reduce or eliminate some of the negative side effects associated with menopause.

Diet—a well-balanced diet can also help balance hormone levels and strengthen your immune system.

Nutritional supplements and/or natural estrogen replacement therapy can also be very helpful with increasing estrogen levels.

Hormone replacement therapy (HRT) involves administering moderate dosages of estrogen, or a combination of estrogen and progesterone, by pill, patch, or cream. HRT treatment will vary from person to person. Consult your physician and have the proper lab tests completed before starting an HRT program.

Andropause and Exercise

Andropause (male menopause) is similar to the hormonal changes that women experience with menopause; however, the symptoms of andropause are not quite as severe as those associated with menopause. Andropause normally occurs between the ages of forty to fifty-five, although it can start as early as age thirty and can last for as long as fifteen to twenty years. It typically involves a gradual decline in the levels of testosterone (unlike menopause, in which there is a sharp drop in estrogen and progesterone). Lack of exercise, poor diet, being overweight, stress, and vasectomy are a few of the variables that can expedite the onset of andropause.

Exercise can help balance your hormones and reduce some of the symptoms. Below is a partial list of the negative side effects of andropause that may be reduced by exercising regularly.

- Decreased testosterone

- Decreased potency

- Decreased sex drive

- Decreased motivation

- Increased fatigue

- Increased irritability

- Increased anxiety

- Increased depression

- Decreased muscle mass

- Decreased muscle strength

- Decreased bone density

- Increased cardiovascular risk

- Increased upper and central body fat

- Increased aging

Exercise can help balance your hormones and reduce some of the symptoms that occur during andropause. Exercising regularly can stimulate the pituitary gland to produce gonadotrophins, which stimulate the testes to produce more testosterone. Weight training and moderate cardiovascular exercise are recommended. Excessive cardiovascular exercise can actually lower testosterone levels. Therefore, exercise should be kept to a moderate level (less than sixty minutes).

Diet—A well balanced diet can also help balance hormone levels. A diet high in protein and low in carbohydrates can help increase muscle mass and maintain strength.

Nutritional supplements and/or natural testosterone replacement therapy can also be very helpful in increasing testosterone levels.

Testosterone replacement therapy (TRT) involves administering moderate dosages of testosterone by injection, pill, patch, or cream. TRT treatment will vary from person to person. Consult your physician and have the proper lab tests completed before starting a TRT program.

Establishing Goals

Without goals, you are like a cork in the ocean, floating wherever the tide wants to take you. You must determine what you what to achieve and how you are going to pursue it. First, you must decide what your own personal goals are. For example, do you want to lose weight, improve muscle tone, or both? Perhaps you are already involved in a particular sport and you would like enhance your performance with an exercise program. Maybe you have a physical illness or injury and need rehabilitation. You might like to get your figure back following a pregnancy. A program can address mental issues such as low self-esteem and depression. Maybe you are just interested in adding some quality years to your life. Your goals might be all of the above. As you can see, everyone will have his or her own reason for creating a personal workout program. When establishing your goals you should make:

- Daily goals

- Weekly goals

- Monthly goals

- Yearly goals

Examples of Goals

Daily Goals

- Increase my leg press by five pounds

- Try out the new cardiovascular machine I haven't used

- Avoid or limit junk food

- Drink at least two extra glasses of water

Weekly Goals

- Complete all three workout days as scheduled

- Add ten minutes to my treadmill routine

- Make it through the entire week of my preplanned diet without cheating

- Show up to the gym at my scheduled time every day

Monthly Goals

- Loose five pounds of fat by the end of the month

- Add an aerobics class to my routine by the end of the month

- Decrease the portion of each meal and stop eating late-night meals

- Take a series of before-and-after pictures and hope to see some progress by the end of the month

Yearly Goals

- Loose at least twenty-five pounds of fat by the end of the year

- Increase my workout schedule from three days a week to five days a week

- Wear my new bathing suit on the beach this summer

- Be in good physical shape for my upcoming high school reunion

- Run in a one- to three-mile charity run

As you can see, there are many different reasons you can use to get yourself motivated. It is up to you to create your own personal list of based upon your own individual goals for improving you physique.

Before-and-After Pictures

It is very difficult to see your body change when you look at yourself every day. Taking before-and-after pictures can be an excellent way to measure the extent of your progress with your exercise program. The before pictures can help motivate you to make the necessary improvements to your physique. The after pictures will allow you to clearly see the progress that you have made over time. I recommend that you take a series of photos approximately every four weeks.

When you take the pictures, you should wear a bathing suit. Also, let the attitude you feel about the current state of your physique show in your posture and your facial expression. Make sure that you get full-frame pictures of your entire body. The pictures you take should include the following poses.

- Front relaxed pose

- Side relaxed pose (left and right)

- Back relaxed pose

Choosing the Proper Atmosphere for Workouts

Choosing the proper atmosphere for your workouts will be a crucial decision. If you are not comfortable with your workout environment, it may destroy your entire exercise program. The following are some options to consider.

- Would you prefer to work out at home?

- Are you interested in your basic local gym?

- Would you prefer a fancy spa atmosphere?

- Does the population of the gym trend more toward young or old people. Does it have more males or females?

Make your choice carefully. If you do not like the atmosphere, you probably will not be motivated to work out.

Choosing Times for Workouts

Once you have determined why you are interested in starting an exercise program, it will be time to list the steps you need to take to complete your goals. The program you design should be based upon your own individual needs. You should ask yourself the following questions:

- How much time will I be willing or able to devote to my workout program?

- How many days a week do I want to work out?

- What particular time of day would I prefer to work out (morning, day, evening)?

- How much time (per day) would I like to workout?

Hiring a Personal Trainer

Personal trainers can be extremely valuable when constructing a workout program. Here is a partial list of what a personal trainer can do for you.

- Educate you on proper gym etiquette

- Help you establish personal goals

- Help you construct an individual workout program

- Instruct you on the proper use of the exercise equipment

- Show you the proper form and technique for individual exercises

- Help motivate you for your workouts

- Spot you on workout equipment

- Help prevent injuries

To ensure good results, choosing a personal trainer should be done carefully. Here are some things to look out for.

- Ask around; who has a good reputation?

- Do they look the part? If they are not in shape, how do they expect to get you into shape?

- Do they have a résumé (a background in the fitness field)?

- Are they certified and insured?

- Are they reliable and dependable?

Bear in mind that I have seen so-called personal trainers who received certification through the mail or by attending a one-day course. I have also known personal trainers who have received their certification through an intense training course but posses very little experience; as a result, they are poor personal trainers. I also know several personal trainers who have no formal certification at all; however, they have tremendous knowledge and are fantastic trainers. Therefore, there is no set rule in making the proper choice. Consider the above-mentioned facts, listen to your instincts, and make your choice wisely.

Personal trainers can be expensive, especially if you use them three or more times a week. If finances are not an issue, that is great! If you are on a budget, I recommend that you use a personal trainer primarily to establish your workout program. Once you feel that you have acquired a sufficient amount of knowledge and feel confident enough to work out alone, it is time to leave the nest and do that. Over time, as you progress through your workouts, you may want to periodically have a session or two with your personal trainer and make some adjustments or add some new exercises.

Having a Training Partner

You may be interested in a training partner. If so, there are some things to consider.

- Do both of you have the same goals?

- Are you both available at the same time on the same day?

- Is your partner reliable and dependable?

- Will your partner be as motivated as you are?

The Advantages of Having a Training Partner

- You can encourage and motivate one another

- You are able to spot and push each other during workouts

- You can analyze one another's physique

The author at Jan Tana Classic Bodybuilding Competition

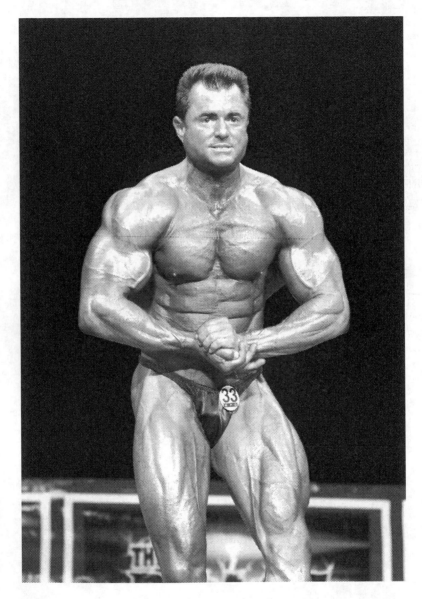

Photo by John Nafpliotis

3

Body Fat

Try not to be too concerned with what the scale says when you weigh yourself. Remember, as you progress with your diet and exercise program, you will lose body fat and gain muscle. Muscle cells are denser tissue than fat cells and fat takes up approximately five times the space of muscle. Because muscle cells are smaller in size than fat cells, a cubic inch of muscle weighs more than a cubic inch fat. Therefore, as you gain muscle and lose fat, your actual weight may not change dramatically, but you should become smaller in size. I recommend that you rely primarily on your instinct when measuring changes in your physique, which can be assisted by asking yourself the following questions.

- How does my physique appear in the mirror?

- How do my clothes fit?

- Do I feel lighter on your feet?

- Does a pinch of skin appear to have less fat?

Body Fat Percentages

Male

- Average body fat for a normal male is 15 to 18 percent

- Body fat for an athletic male is under 13 percent

- Body fat for a lean male is under 11 percent

- Body fat for a male at cardiovascular risk is over 18 percent

- Current average body fat for a U. S. male is 22 percent

Female

- Average body fat for a normal female is 25 to 27 percent

- Body fat for an athletic female is under 23 percent

- Body fat for a lean female is under 19 percent

- Body fat for a female at cardiovascular risk is over 27 percent

- Current average body fat for a U. S. female is 35 percent

Measuring Body Fat

It is a good idea to have your body fat tested at different intervals throughout your exercise program. This will help indicate specific results as you progress. There are several methods for testing body fat, and keep in mind that some methods are more accurate than others are. I recommend using the same method of body-fat testing throughout your program to maintain consistent measurements of changes as they occur.

There are several factors to consider when choosing a method for calculating the percentage of body fat, also called body composition: cost, availability, and accuracy. Starting with the least accurate method first, the following is a list of the most common methods used for determining the percent of individual body fat.

Height–weight tables—This is a chart. You find your height on one axis and follow along on the other until you find your weight. Unfortunately, this method is inaccurate due to the fact that it does not take into consideration the difference between lean muscle mass and body composition.

Skinfold measurements—This method uses a tool called a skinfold caliper. Gyms, health clubs, and wellness centers most commonly use this method. You could opt to purchase one of your own; they are inexpensive and easy to use. You can take the measurements yourself, but it is easier for someone else to take them for you. Make sure that the same person takes the measurements each time to help ensure accuracy. The skinfold caliper is used to measure subcutaneous tissue (tissue beneath the skin) in from three to seven sites on the body. Accuracy is to within 3 percent (plus or minus) with this method.

Bioelectrical impedance analysis (BIA)—To get a BIA, you stand barefoot on a scale that calculates your body fat in a matter of seconds. It uses a low-voltage current of electricity, which travels up one leg and down the other. Fat, being a poor conductor of electricity, causes resistance to the current. This resistance is measured and the percentage of body fat estimated. Today many gyms, health clubs, and wellness centers have these machines. Accuracy is approximately 3 percent (plus or minus). The following is a list of several factors that can manipulate the accuracy of this test.

- Not eating or drinking within four hours of the test

- Not exercising within twelve hours of the test

- Urinating completely before the test

- Alcohol consumption within forty-eight hours of the test

- Taking diuretics prior to taking the test

Hydrostatic weighing (underwater weighing)—Hydrostatic weighing is regarded as the "gold standard" for testing body fat percentage because it is known to be the most accurate: approximately plus or minus 1 percent. The process requires an individual to be submerged in a tank of water. Lean body mass (bone, muscle, and connective tissue) sinks, while body fat floats. Fat mass will make a body lighter in water, indicating a higher percentage of body fat. Here is a list of disadvantages of the hydrostatic weighing method.

- It can be expensive

- It can be hard to find a location for the test

- Testing is time consuming

- In-depth knowledge is required to administer the test

- Some people find being submerged in a tank difficult or uncomfortable

The following is a list of less common methods used for testing body fat percentage. They can be both costly and hard to find.

Bod pod (air displacement)—approximately 3 percent (plus or minus) accuracy

Dual X-ray absorptionmetry (DEXA)—accuracy N/A

Near inferred interactance (NIR) Futrex 5000—accuracy N/A

Whichever method you choose, I recommend using the metohd and the same person to administer it each time you test. This will allow for both consistency and accuracy in recording changes in your body fat.

Calculating Lean Body Mass

If have successfully determined body-fat percentage, you will be able to calculate your body lean mass (muscle weight) and fat weight. Here is an example of how to do it.

- Starting with 150 pounds (scale weight), subtract 30 percent (body fat percentage) = 105 lbs (lean body mass weight)

- Starting with 150 pounds (scale weight), subtract 105 lbs (lean body mass weight) = 45 lbs (fat weight)

If you set your goal to be 20 percent body fat at 150 pounds, you would need to drop an additional 15 pounds of body fat weight, as illustrated below.

- 150 lbs (scale weight), subtract 20 percent (body fat percentage) = 120 lbs (lean body mass weight)

- 150 lbs (scale weight), subtract 120 lbs (lean body mass weight) = 30 lbs (fat weight)

The author at a photo shoot for MuscleTech

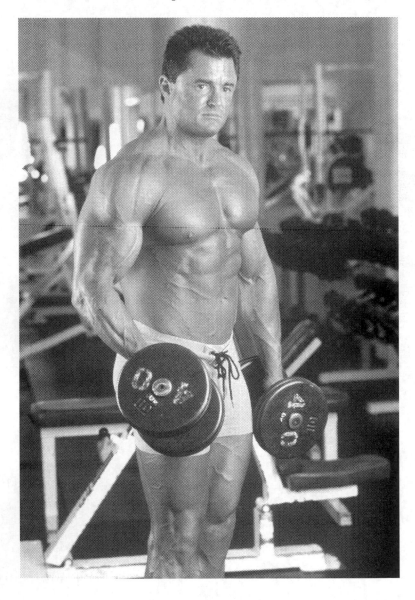

Photo by Mitsuru Okabe (www.mocvideo.com)

4

Muscle Anatomy

Muscle Types

The human body possesses three different types of muscles: skeletal (striated), heart (cardiac), and smooth (visceral).

Skeletal Muscle

Skeletal muscle consists of striated muscle groups attached to tendons and bones. The contraction of skeletal muscle is voluntary and is responsible for movements such as walking and lifting. Skeletal muscle *can* become fatigued.

Heart Muscle

Heart muscle is made up of striated muscle cells branched together that contract in synchronization. Heart muscle is usually an involuntary muscle. The heart (cardiac) needs to be exercised just as other the muscles of your body (skeletal muscle) need exercise to maintain good condition. This is where the term cardiovascular exercise comes from.

Smooth Muscle

Smooth muscles are found in the walls of hollow organs such as the blood vessels, throat, and intestines. When contracted they regulate movement within these structures. Smooth muscle is also an involuntary muscle, and cannot become fatigued.

Muscle Fiber Types

Skeletal muscle is generally composed of two different types of muscle fibers: slow-twitch muscle fibers and fast-twitch muscle fibers.

Slow Twitch

Slow-twitch (type I) muscle fibers have long muscle fibers that contract slow and steadily for low-intensity, high-endurance activities. Slow-twitch muscle fibers are highly resistant to fatigue and are primarily used for aerobic activities such as long distance running and daily life activities. Slow-twitch muscle fibers are high in myoglobin, making them "red meat."

Fast Twitch

Fast-twitch (type II) muscle fibers have short muscle fibers that contract quickly for short, explosive bursts of power; they are efficient for high-intensity, low-endurance activities. Fast-twitch muscle fibers fatigue quickly and are primarily used for anaerobic activities such as sprinting and weight lifting. Slow-twitch muscle fibers are low in myoglobin, making them "white meat." Fast-twice muscle can also be broken down into two separate categories (type II A) and (type II B).

Fast Twitch (Type II A)

Fast-twitch (type II A) muscles are good for extended anaerobic activities such as sprinting 400 meters or swimming a 50-meter race. They posses numerous blood capillaries and do not fatigue as quickly as type II B.

Fast Twitch (Type II B)

Fast-twitch (type II B) muscles are efficient in extremely short anaerobic activities such as 50- to 100-meter sprints and heavy weight lifting. They posses a small number of capillaries and fatigue very quickly.

Every individual has a different number of each type of muscle: some people have 50 percent of each type and others possess a larger percentage of one of the types. The percentages of different muscle fibers are determined genetically before birth; however, there is some evidence that endurance athletes tend to develop a greater number of slow-twitch muscle fibers and power athletes tend to develop a greater number of fast-twitch muscle fibers.

Muscle Contraction Types

Skeletal muscle possesses three types of muscle contractions: isotonic, isokinetic, and isometric.

Isotonic

Isotonic contraction is the most common type of muscle contraction. It refers to the shortening of the muscle as it contracts. For example, during a bicep curl the bicep muscles contract against gravity and shorten, lifting the forearm toward the upper arm. (Isotonic contractions are sometimes referred to as concentric or eccentric contractions.)

Isokinetic

Isokinetic contraction is similar to isotonic, with the muscle fiber shortening. However, it requires constant speed throughout the entire range of motion: for example, an arm stroke when swimming. (Isokinetic contractions are sometimes referred to as concentric or eccentric contractions.)

Isometric

Isometric contraction refers to a muscle contracting against an immovable object: for example, trying to lift a fixed object. Another example would be pushing your palms against each other without movement or range of motion. (Isometric contractions are sometimes referred to as static contractions.)

Muscular Anatomy Chart (Front)

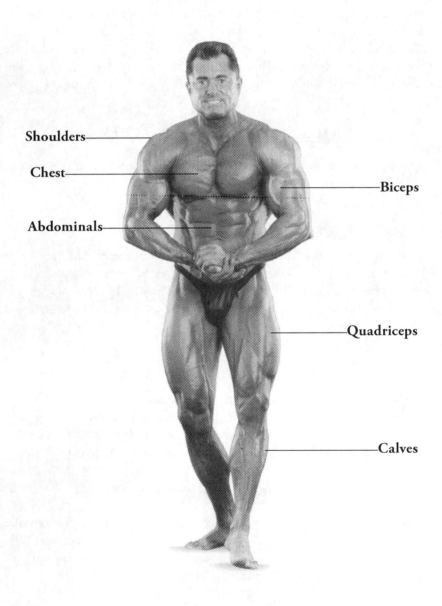

Shoulders

Chest

Biceps

Abdominals

Quadriceps

Calves

Muscular Anatomy Chart
(Back)

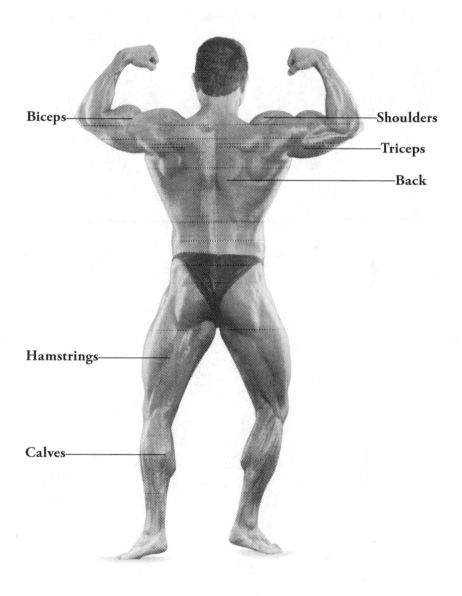

Biceps

Shoulders

Triceps

Back

Hamstrings

Calves

5

Constructing a Workout Program

Consulting Your Physician

It is a good idea to consult your physician or health care provider prior to starting any exercise program. This list contains reasons you might want to do so.

- Pre-existing cardiac (heart) condition—heart attack, clogged arteries, bypass surgery

- Pre-existing respiratory condition—bronchitis, asthma, emphysema

- Pre-existing osteoporosis condition— decreased bone density

- Pre-existing injured back—sciatica, herniated disk, fractured vertebra

- Previous stroke—impaired blood supply to the brain

- Previous operation—knee, shoulder, or hip surgery

- The use of certain medications

- Hypertension (high blood pressure)

Blood Pressure Ranges

Systolic = Heart Beating	Diastolic = Heart Resting
120 = First Number	80 = Second Number

Blood Pressure Ranges	Classification
100/60 to 120/80	Optimal
120/80 to 140/90	Prehypertension
140/90 and above	High blood pressure

Studies conducted; show that increased risk of cardiovascular disease is clearly linked to *systolic* high blood pressure hypertension. (when measurement taken at rest).

Note: (When exercising, the systolic number goes up)

Eating Prior to Exercising

When you eat food, the body begins the process of digestion and absorption. During digestion, the body directs blood flow to the stomach and internal organs. When you exercise, blood is redirected away from the stomach and internal organs in order to be utilized by the muscles. The redirection of blood to the muscles can cause early fatigue during exercise.

The length of time for digestion and absorption depends on the type and quantity of food. Normally fat, protein, and fiber take longer to digest. In addition, large quantities of food take longer to digest. For example, meal replacement shakes digest faster than solid foods. As general a rule, eat a small meal at least one to two hours before exercising, and wait two to three hours for larger meals. Approximately 50 percent of heart attacks occur after eating a heavy meal.

Workout Gear

Workout gear includes attire and various other items that can enhance your workouts. When working out, you should always wear loose-fitting clothes that are comfortable. Sweats and stretch clothes are generally suitable. A good pair of sneakers is also important, especially if you plan to incorporate cardiovascular exercise into your exercise program.

If you will be traveling to a gym, I recommend bringing a gym bag or a small backpack to carry additional items. The following is a list of optional items you may want to consider bringing with you.

- Water bottle (to prevent dehydration)

- Workout gloves (to protect hands and prevent them from slipping)

- Weight-lifting belt (to protect lower back)

- Towel (for sweating, showering, covering pads, and benches or showering)

- Workout logbook (to record daily workout program)

- Protein shake, bar, or some fruit (in case you get hungry)

- Spare clothes (to change out of sweaty cloths)

- Walkman/radio (to listen to your own music)

- Book or magazine (to read while performing cardiovascular exercise)

Proper Gym Etiquette

- Do not bang or drop weights

- Put all weights and equipment away when you are finished using them

- Wipe down equipment and benches after using them

- Be courteous and share equipment with other members

The Program Outline

After you have decided how much time you are willing to allocate to your workouts, you will be ready to design the specifics. To begin, you should always warm up prior to exercising. After that, your exercise program can be divided into two parts: **Weight training** (anaerobic muscular conditioning) and **cardiovascular exercise** (aerobic conditioning). If your goals are focused on trimming body fat and losing weight, a larger percentage of your workout should entail cardiovascular exercise, with less emphasis on weight training. If you are more interested in toning, reshaping, or building your muscles, your workout should include more weight training and less cardiovascular exercise.

Warming up

Warming up before workouts increases your body temperature. It also increases the blood flow to your heart, lungs, muscles, and soft tissue; this includes the ligaments, tendons, and cartilage. Warming up prepares the body for exercise and helps prevent injuries from occurring.

Warm-up Techniques

Stretching before you begin exercising is essential. Light cardiovascular exercise can be used as a warm-up: treadmill, cycling, et cetera. Start slowly and progress gradually. At the beginning of your workouts you should warm up with high repetitions and light weight on the first couple of sets.

The author at a photo shoot for MuscleTech

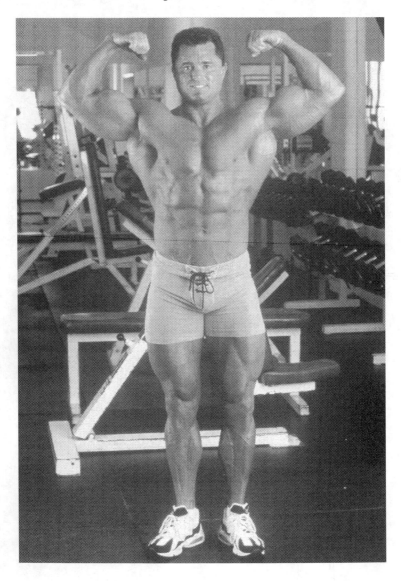

Photo by Mitsuru Okabe (www.mocvideo.com)

6

Stretching

Stretching can be performed before, during, and after an exercise. Some of the benefits of stretching are listed below.

Benefits of Stretching for Exercise

- Stimulates fresh blood and oxygen moving to joints and muscles from overexertion

- Increases flexibility and range of motion (ROM)

- Warms up muscles prior to exercise

- Helps minimize risk of injuries

- Helps reduce post-workout soreness

Basic Stretching Techniques

Upper-Body Stretch

Photography by Lon Miller

Straight Bar Stretch

(Shoulders, Chest, Back, Biceps, and Triceps)

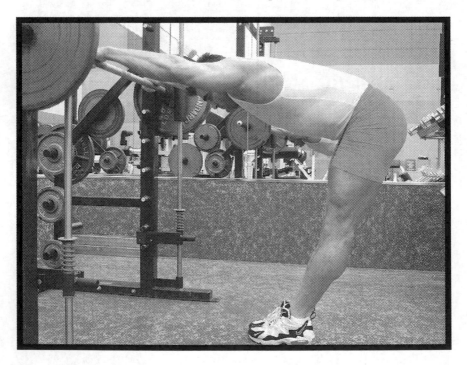

Straight Bar Stretch

(Shoulders, Chest, Back, Biceps, and Triceps)

- Position a barbell at approximately shoulder height and grasp the bar with an overhand grip approximately shoulder width apart

- Stand with feet together several feet from the bar

- Lean back using your body weight and bring your hips behind your feet (try to keep your torso parallel to the floor)

- Hold the stretch for approximately 20 to 30 seconds and repeat several times

Upper-Body Stretch

Hanging Bar Stretch

(Shoulders, Chest, Back, Biceps, and Triceps)

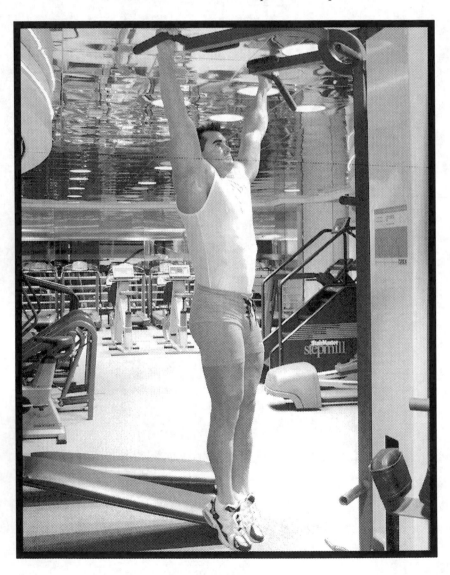

Hanging Bar Stretch
(Shoulders, Chest, Back, Biceps, and Triceps)

- Grasp a pull-up bar with an overhand grip approximately shoulder width apart

- Allow your body to hang off the ground in a relaxed position for 20 to 30 seconds and repeat several times

Lower-Body Stretch

Lunge Stretch

(Quadriceps, Hamstrings, and Calves)

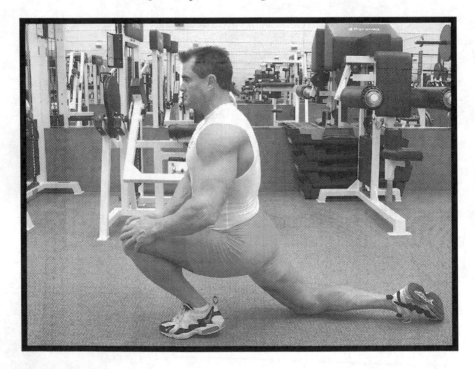

Lunge Stretch

(*Quadriceps, Hamstrings, and Calves*)

- Step forward with your left foot in a lunge position while keeping your right leg stretched behind you, resting your knee on the floor

- Place your hands on your left knee for support

- Hold the stretch for 20 to 30 seconds and repeat several times

- Next, do the same for your right leg

Lower-Body Stretch

Achilles Stretch

(Achilles Tendons, Hamstrings, and Calves)

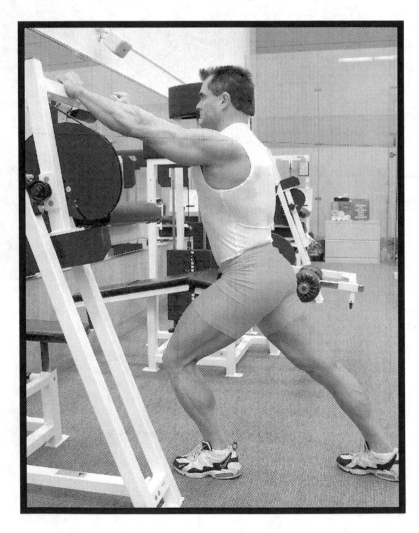

Achilles Stretch
(*Achilles Tendons, Hamstrings, and Calves*)

- Using your arms, rest your body weight on a solid surface (wall or bar) approximately shoulder-width apart

- Step in front of your hips with your left leg and slightly bend your knee

- Step backward behind your hips with your right leg, keeping it straight with your heel planted flat on the floor (the further you step backward with your right leg the deeper the stretch will be)

- Hold the stretch for 20 to 30 seconds and repeat several times

- Next, do the same for your right leg

The author at a photo shoot for MuscleMag

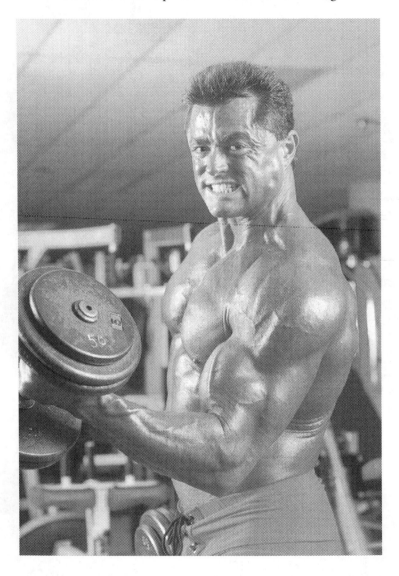

Photo by Ralph DeHaan (www.ralphdehaan.com)

7

Weight Training
(*Muscular Conditioning*)

Weight training is considered anaerobic exercise. Anaerobic exercise requires less oxygen then aerobic conditioning and involves a shorter duration of time with a higher level of intensity. Anaerobic conditioning usually pertains to activities such as weight lifting. The primary focus is on improving muscle tone, shape, and strength. Weight Training can also be referred to as weight lifting, resistance training, muscular conditioning, and anaerobic exercise.

Examples of Weight-Training Exercises

Weight training includes any type of resistance to weight: for example, free weights, weight machines, or resistance to your own body weight.

- Barbell bench press (free weight)

- Leg extension (weight machine)

- Pull-up (body weight)

Benefits of Weight Training

- Contributes to the health of your heart muscle and blood vessels

- Increases the efficiency of your lungs and pumps more oxygen through your body

- Increases circulations throughout your entire body

- Increases metabolism

- Burns calories (reduces body fat)

- Improves the quality of muscle tone

- Helps improve sleep

The benefits of weight training are similar to the ones listed under benefits of cardiovascular exercise. However, with weight training you can isolate and accentuate the quality of individual muscle groups or body parts. This allows you to sculpt your body into a shape that you desire.

Reps and Sets

- A repetition, or "rep" for short, is one complete exercise movement from start to finish

- A set is a group of repetitions

- For example, two sets of bench press for twelve reps of bench press = 2 x 12

Recommended Reps and Sets

- Two to three different exercises per muscle group or "body part"

- Two to four sets per individual exercise

- Eight to fifteen repetitions per set

Determining How Much Weight

Let your body dictate how much weight is necessary for individual exercises. For example, if your goal is to perform ten repetitions and you can only do six, the weight you are using is too heavy. On the other hand, if your goal is to perform ten repetitions and you can do fifteen, the weight you are using is too light. As you progress through your workouts, you will use this method to decide when to increase the weight.

Exercise Larger Muscle Groups First

As a rule you should exercise larger muscle groups first (chest, back, shoulders, quadriceps, and hamstrings) and smaller groups second (biceps, Tricep, calves, and abdominals). Smaller muscle groups generally support the action of larger muscle groups. If you fatigue a smaller muscle before exercising a larger one, you will significantly decrease the potential weight and or reps for larger body parts; therefore exercising smaller muscle groups first will compromise the intensity of training larger ones. For example, do not exercise your Tricep before exercising your chest.

Exercise Muscles from Different Angles

To develop a muscle most efficiently, you will need to train it from several different angles. To be most effective, you will need to choose several different exercises for each individual muscle. For example, when you exercise your chest do a flat bench press, an incline bench press, and chest flye exercise. (Individual weight-training exercises discussed the following chapter).

Priority Training

Priority Training involves focusing on one particular muscle group. This allows you to contour your workout based on your own individual needs. For example, if your upper body is naturally in better condition than your lower body, you may want to priority train your legs. You can do this by placing a larger percentage of your weight training on your legs. Perhaps you are content with most of your body; however, you feel you have one or two body parts that require more attention. You can give priority to training these individual areas.

Creating Illusions

You can create any body shape you desire with weight training. You can also create illusions by isolating and enhancing specific groups. If your goal is to have a smaller-looking waist and hips, you can tone and shape your shoulder and lat muscles. This will create the illusion that your waist and hips are slimmer. I know many girls who feel that their legs look too large. Developing more muscle on their upper bodies can create the illusion that they are more proportionally balanced.

Basic Weight-Training Techniques

- Your weight-training program should include a combination of free weights, weighted machines, and body weight (weighted machines have a variety of adjustments to accommodate various body types)

- Always exhale when exerting the maximum amount of force during an exercise

- Use smooth, controlled movements; do not jerk the weights

- Concentrate on using proper form and technique and it will become a habit

- Concentrate and focus strictly on the muscle you are working

- During each rep you should raise or lower the weight for approximately 1 to 2 seconds, and flex the muscles you are working at the peak of the movement, then raise or lower the weight for approximately 1 to 2 seconds

- Apply approximately 60 seconds of rest between sets (rest period)

- Use higher repetitions with lower weights to tone and shape muscles (over 12 repetitions)

- Use lower repetitions with heavier weights to build larger muscle. 8 to 12 reps is the optimal number for gains in strength, shape, tone, and size, (for the beginner I do not recommend using a weight that you can only lift for six repetitions or less)

- If you experience unusual pain during exercise, stop the exercise or lower the repetitions

- Adjust weight machines to fit your specific body type so that you obtain the proper range of motion (ROM) without putting unneeded stress on joints (adjust seats, pads, pulleys, etc.)

Workout Tips

Over time your body may grow accustomed to your workout regime, therefore your progress may begin to slow down or plateau. You can stimulate your workouts by shocking your muscles using different techniques for a couple of weeks.

- Change the variation of exercises for each body part, or cardiovascular movement.

- Change the number of repetitions for each set. If you have been doing 12 to 15 repetitions switch to 8 to 10 with a heaver weight, or increase the intensity of your cardiovascular exercise for a shorter duration.

You are in control of developing your own workout program. When constructing your program, try to choose weight training and cardiovascular exercises that are fun and that interest you. If you do, your workouts will not seem like a chore.

Note: Your potential for progress in increasing both strength and muscle tone is greater at the beginning of your weight-training program. Someone who has never trained may acquire very rapid results and then plateau. For example, in the first ten weeks of training you may gain up to 25 percent in strength, shape, tone, and size; in the following ten weeks you may only attain up to 5 percent gains. A person who has consistently been training for a long period of time may see slow but sure, gradual progress.

The author at a photo shoot for MuscleTech

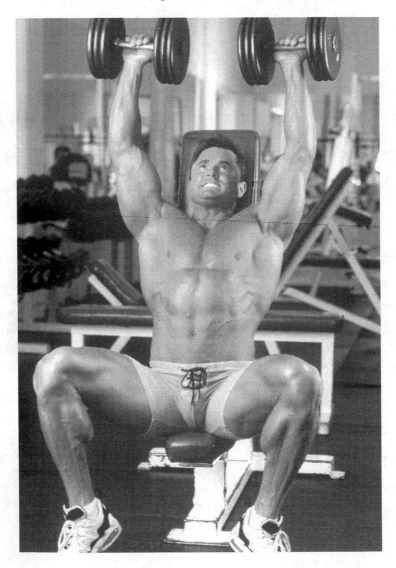

Photo by Mitsuru Okabe (www.mocvideo.com)

8

Basic Weight-Training Exercises

If you choose to join a gym or health club, there should be a qualified instructor to show you the proper use of the exercise equipment. Another option is to hire a personal trainer, as discussed earlier in this book. The following is a list of basic weight-training exercises listed by individual muscle groups.

Upper Body

Chest

- Barbell Flat Bench Chest Press
- Dumbbell Incline Chest Press
- Chest Machine Flyes

Back

- Seated Wide-grip Straight-bar Cable Pull-downs
- Seated V-grip Cable Rows
- Dumbbell One-arm Rows

Shoulders

- Dumbbell Overhead Shoulders Press
- Dumbbell Seated Side Lateral Raises
- Dumbbell Standing Bent-over Lateral Raises

Biceps

- Barbell Standing Bicep Curls
- Dumbbell Seated Bicep Curls
- Cable Machine Bicep Curls

Tricep

- Barbell Lying Tricep Extensions
- Cable Machine Tricep Pushdowns
- Dumbbell Tricep Extensions

Abdominals

- Crunches
- Decline Sit-ups
- Seated Bent-knee Leg Raises

Lower Body

Quadriceps

- Barbell Leg Squats
- Leg Machine Press
- Leg Machine Extensions

Hamstrings

- Barbell Straight-leg Dead Lifts
- Lying Machine Leg Curls
- Dumbbell Lunges

Calves

- Barbell Standing Calf Raises
- Seated Machine Calf Raises
- Dumbbell Standing Calf Raises

Refer to chapter, (7) for methods to determine how much weight to use for individual exercises.

Description of Individual Exercises

Upper-Body Exercises

(Photography by Lon Miller)

Chest

Barbell Flat Bench Chest Press

Start/Finish

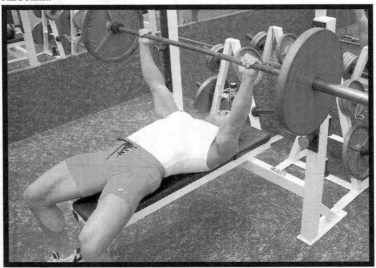

Midpoint

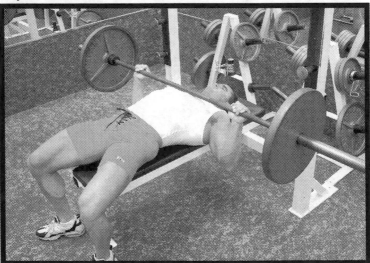

Chest

Barbell Flat Bench Chest Press

Starting Position:

- Lie on your back on a flat bench

- Grasp the barbell with your hands slightly wider than shoulder-width apart

- Remove the barbell from the rack and position the bar over your chest with arms fully extended upward

Movement:

- Slowly lower the weight to the middle of your chest

- Keep elbows outward from your torso

- Raise the weight back to the starting position and flex your chest muscles

- Slowly lower the weight; repeat for the desired number of repetitions

Chest

Dumbbell Incline Chest Press

Start/Finish

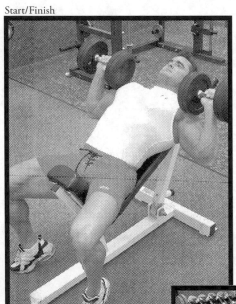

Midpoint

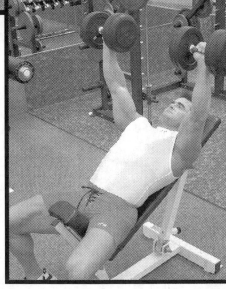

Chest

Dumbbell Incline Chest Press

Starting Position:

- Adjust the back pad on the bench to approximately a 45-degree angle

- Sit on the bench, grasp one dumbbell with each hand, and place them on your thighs

- Lean back and swing the dumbbells upward one at a time, bringing them just above your shoulders

Movement:

- Raise the dumbbells upward overhead until your arms are fully extended and flex your chest muscles

- Slowly lower the weight; repeat for the desired number of repetitions

Chest

Chest Machine Flyes

Start/Finish

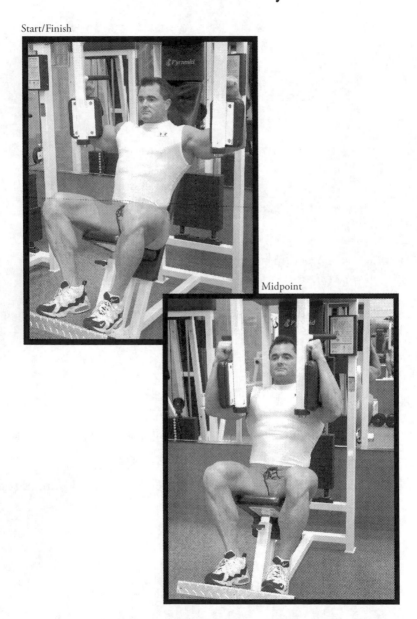

Midpoint

Chest

Chest Machine Flyes

Starting Position:

- Sit on the bench with your head and back resting against the back pad

- Adjust the seat height so that your upper arms are parallel to the floor while your forearms are pushing against the pads

Movement:

- Exert pressure on the pads from your forearms, keeping your elbows below your forearms

- Continue to exert force until the arm pads come together in front of you and flex your chest muscles

- Slowly return to the starting position while resisting the weight; repeat for the desired number of repetitions

Back

Seated Wide-grip Straight-bar Cable Pull-downs

Start/Finish

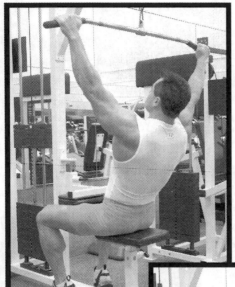

Midpoint

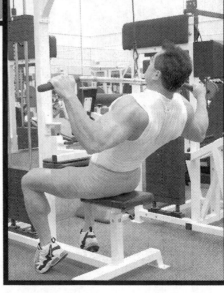

Back

Seated Wide-grip Straight-bar Cable Pull-downs

Starting Position:

- Sit facing the cable pull-down machine

- Lock your knees under the pads

- Grasp the bar with an overhand grip, hands slightly wider than shoulder-width apart

Movement:

- Pull the bar down to the top of your chest and flex your back muscles

- Slowly allow your arms to straighten and return to the starting position while resisting the weight; repeat for the desired number of repetitions

Back

Seated V-grip Cable Rows

Start/Finish

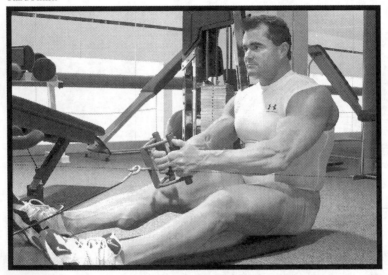

Midpoint

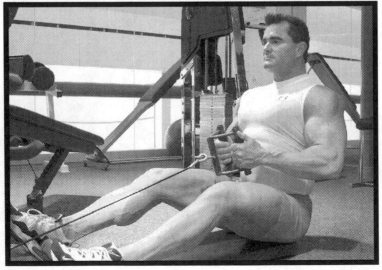

Back

Seated V-grip Cable Rows

Starting Position:

- Sit on the pad facing the low-row cable machine

- Secure your feet against the apparatus and grasp the v-grip bar

Movement:

- Keep your knees slightly bent and pull the bar toward your midsection; hold and flex your back muscles

- Slowly allow your arms to straighten and return to the starting position while resisting the weight; repeat for the desired number of repetitions

Back

Dumbbell One-arm Rows

Start/Finish

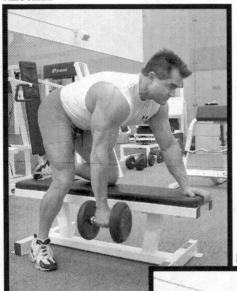

Midpoint

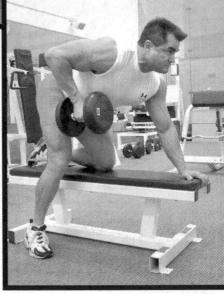

Back

Dumbbell One-arm Rows

Starting Position:

- Place your right foot on the floor and left knee and left arm on the bench

- Your body weight should be on your left arm and knee and your torso should be parallel to the floor with your head and chest facing forward

Movement:

- Grasp a dumbbell with your right hand, pull it toward your shoulder until it is even with your torso, and flex your back muscles

- Slowly lower the dumbbell while resisting the weight

- After you have completed your desired number of repetitions, repeat the same movement with your left side

Shoulders

Dumbbell Overhead Shoulder Press

Start/Finish

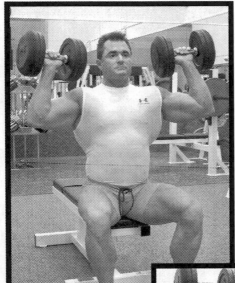

Midpoint

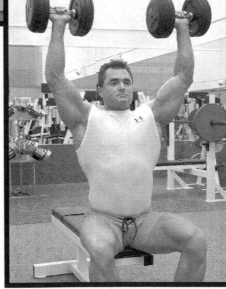

Shoulders

Dumbbell Overhead Shoulder Press

Starting Position:

- Sit on a flat bench and grasp one dumbbell with each hand

- Swing the dumbbells up to your shoulders, keeping your elbows at your sides and your palms facing forward

Movement:

- Push the dumbbells upward until your arms are straight over your head

- Slowly lower your arms to the starting position while resisting the weight; repeat for the desired number of repetitions

Shoulders

Dumbbell Side Lateral Raises

Start/Finish

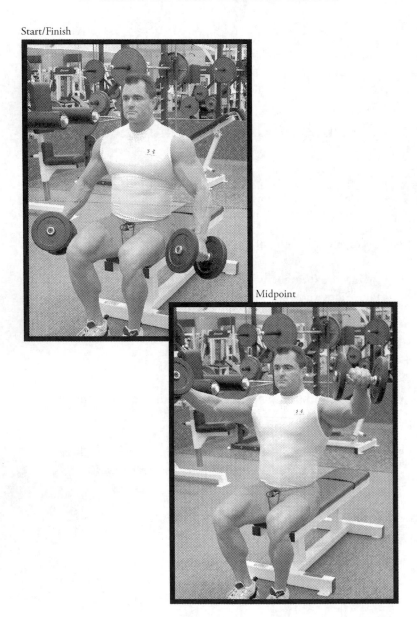

Midpoint

Shoulders

Dumbbell Side Lateral Raises

Starting Position:

- Sit on a flat bench and grasp one dumbbell with each hand

- Bend your elbows slightly with your palms facing your body

Movement:

- Raise the dumbbells upward (do not swing them) to approximately eye level with your palms facing the floor and flex your shoulder muscles

- Slowly lower the dumbbells back to the starting position while resisting the weight; repeat for the desired number of repetitions

Shoulders

Dumbbell Bent-over Laterals

Start/Finish

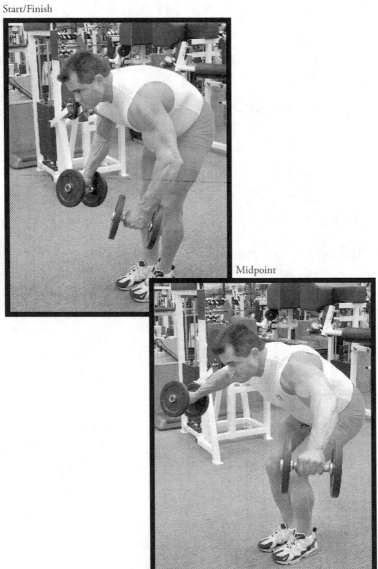

Midpoint

Shoulders

Dumbbell Bent-over Laterals

Starting Position:

- Grasp one dumbbell in each hand, standing with your feet approximately shoulder-width apart

- Bend over so that your torso is parallel to the floor and let the dumbbells hang, keeping a slight bend in your elbows with your palms facing each other

Movement:

- Raise the dumbbells apart (do not swing them) toward the ceiling until they are approximately even with your torso and flex your shoulder muscles

- Slowly lower the dumbbells back to the starting position while resisting the weight; repeat for the desired number of repetitions

Biceps

Barbell Standing Bicep Curls

Start/Finish

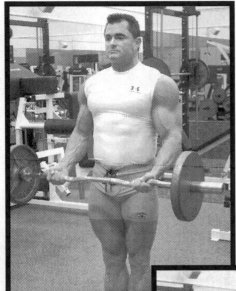

Midpoint

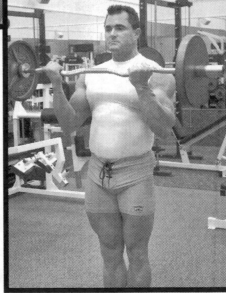

Biceps

Barbell Standing Bicep Curls

Starting Position:

- Stand with your legs together or up to shoulder-width apart

- Grasp the desired barbell with your palms facing upward, with hands approximately shoulder-width apart and elbows to your sides

Movement:

- Curl (do not swing barbell) the bar upward until it is under your chin and flex your bicep muscles

- Slowly lower the barbell back to the starting position while resisting the weight; repeat for the desired number of repetitions

Biceps

Dumbbell Seated Bicep Curls

Start/Finish

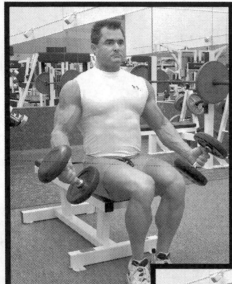

Midpoint

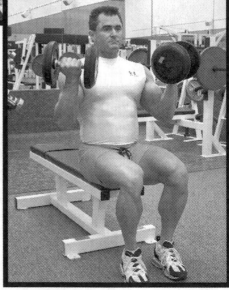

Biceps

Dumbbell Seated Bicep Curls

Starting Position:

- Sit on a flat bench with your feet close together and grasp one dumbbell in each hand

- Hang dumbbells at your sides with your palms facing upward

Movement:

- Curl dumbbells upward (do not swing them) until they are under your chin and flex your bicep muscles

- Slowly lower the barbell back to the starting position while resisting the weight; repeat for the desired number of repetitions

Biceps

Cable Machine Bicep Curls

Start/Finish

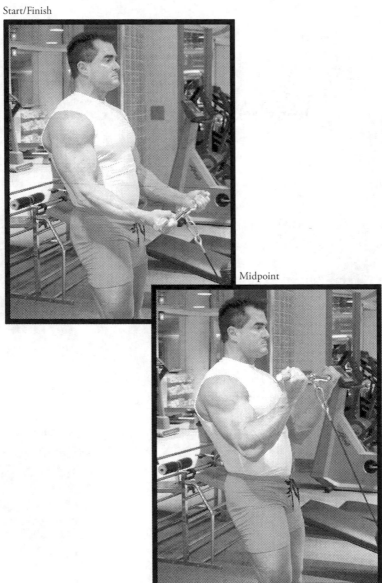

Midpoint

Biceps

Cable Machine Bicep Curls

Starting Position:

- Stand with your legs together or up to shoulder width-apart

- Grasp the desired bar with your palms facing upward, with hands approximately shoulder-width apart and elbows to your sides

Movement:

- Curl (do not swing bar) the bar upward until it is under your chin and flex your bicep muscles

- Slowly lower the barbell back to the starting position while resisting the weight; repeat for the desired number of repetitions

Triceps

Barbell Lying Tricep Extensions

Start/Finish

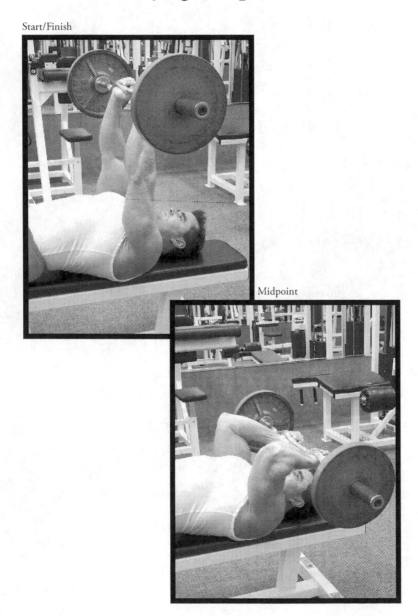

Midpoint

Triceps

Barbell Lying Tricep Extensions

Starting Position:

- Lying on your back on a bench, grasp the desired barbell with your hands slightly closer than shoulder width apart and stretch your arms and the barbell toward the ceiling

Movement:

- Slowly bend your elbows, lowering the weight toward your forehead (keep your upper arms vertical and your elbows facing the ceiling)

- Raise the weight back to the starting position and flex your tricep muscles; repeat for the desired number of repetitions

Triceps

Cable Machine Tricep Push-downs

Start/Finish

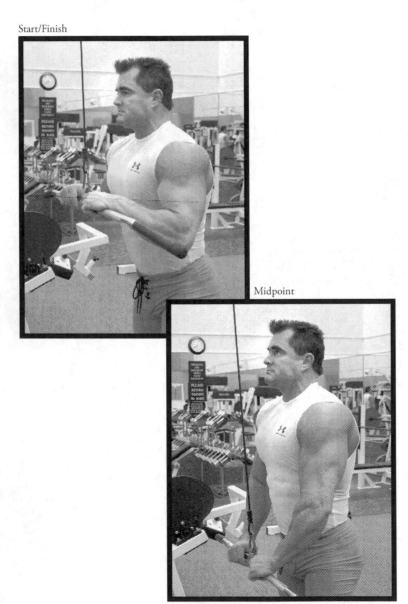

Midpoint

Triceps

Cable Machine Tricep Push-downs

Starting Position:

- Grasp the bar on the cable machine with your hands slightly closer than shoulder-width apart; your palms face toward the floor and your forearms are slightly above parallel to the floor

Movement:

- Push the bar downward toward the floor until your arms are straight and flex your tricep muscles

- Raise the weight back to the starting position; repeat for the desired number of repetitions

Triceps

Dumbbell Tricep Extensions

Start/Finish

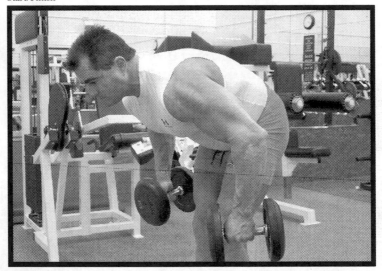

Midpoint

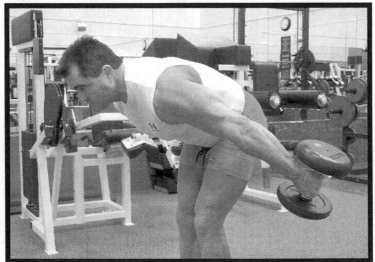

Triceps

Dumbbell Tricep Extensions

Starting Position:

- Stand with your feet together and bend forward at your hips so that your torso is parallel to the floor

- Grasp one dumbbell with each hand, keeping your upper arms tucked to your sides parallel with your torso

Movement:

- Slowly raise the lower part of your arm toward the ceiling until your arms are straight and flex your tricep muscles

- Slowly lower the dumbbells back to the starting position; repeat for the desired number of repetitions

Abdominals

Crunches

Start/Finish

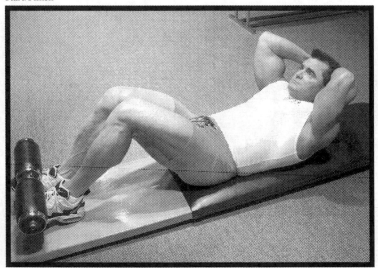

Midpoint

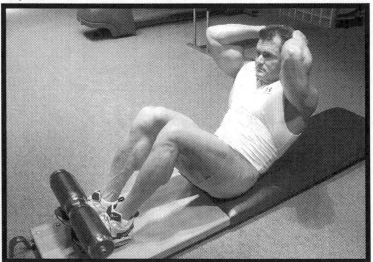

Abdominals

Crunches

Starting Position:

- Lie on a flat sit-up bench and tuck your feet under the foot pads, keeping your knees bent

- Position your hands behind your head or on your chest

Movement:

- Lift your shoulders several inches off the bench while flexing your abdominal muscles throughout the entire movement

- Slowly lower back to the starting position; repeat for the desired number of repetitions

Abdominals

Decline Sit-ups

Start/Finish

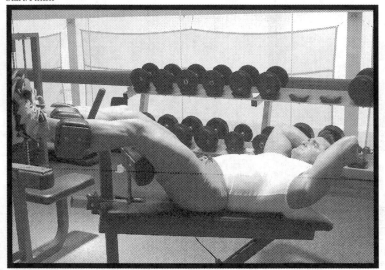

Midpoint

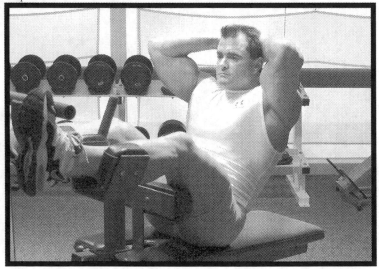

Abdominals

Decline Sit-ups

Starting Position:

- Lie on a decline bench and tuck your feet under the foot pads

- Position your hands behind your head or on your chest

Movement:

- Lift your shoulders off the bench and bring your torso toward your upper legs while flexing your abdominal muscles throughout the entire movement

- Slowly lower your torso, but do not go all the way back to the bench with your shoulders (stop at approximately a 45-degree angle); repeat for the desired number of repetitions

Abdominals

Seated Bent-knee Leg Raises

Start/Finish

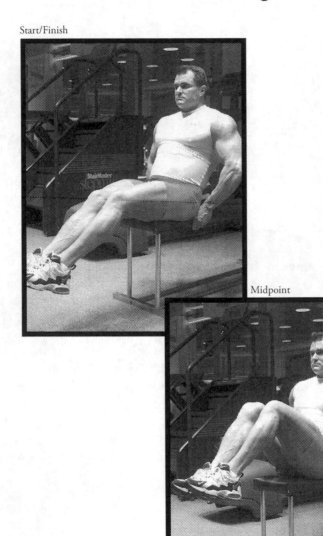

Midpoint

Abdominals

Seated Bent-knee Leg Raises

Starting Position:

- Sit on a bench and grasp the bench behind your lower back

- Position your torso at approximately a 45-degree angle leaning backward

Movement:

- Slowly lift your legs upward while bending your knees, bringing your upper legs toward your torso

- Make sure that you flex your abdominal muscles throughout the entire movement

- Slowly straighten your legs back to the starting position; repeat for the desired number of repetitions

Lower-Body Exercises

Quadriceps

Barbell Leg Squats

Start/Finish

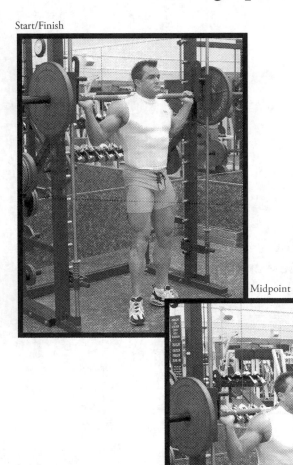

Midpoint

Quadriceps

Barbell Leg Squats

Starting Position:

- Place the barbell behind your neck on your shoulders (trap muscles)

- Grip the bar with your hands slightly wider than shoulder-width apart and your palms facing forward

- Position your feet slightly wider than shoulder-width apart

- Keep your back straight and your head and chest up without leaning forward throughout the entire movement

Movement:

- Slowly bend your knees and lower the weight until your upper legs are parallel to the floor

- Slowly straighten your legs, driving the weight upward back to the starting position and flex your quadricep muscles; repeat for the desired number of repetitions

Quadriceps

Leg Machine Press

Start/Finish

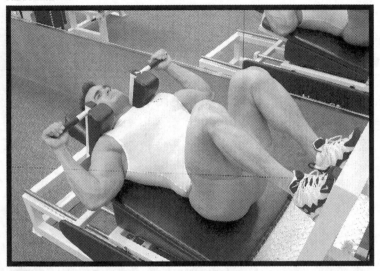

Midpoint

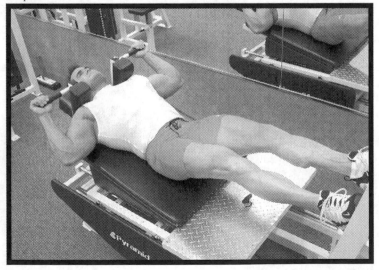

Quadriceps

Leg Machine Press

Starting Position:

- Lie on the leg press machine and adjust the position of the seat

- Your knees should be bent with your upper legs close to your chest, your feet should be placed together or up to shoulder-width apart on the weight platform, and your hands should be grasping the handles attached to the seat

Movement:

- Slowly straighten your legs, driving the weight upward and flex your quadricep muscles

- Slowly bend your knees and lower the weight back to the starting position; repeat for the desired number of repetitions

Note: Some leg press machines start with your legs in the straight position

Quadriceps

Leg Machine Extensions

Start/Finish

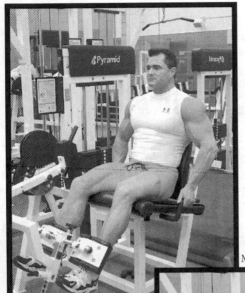

Midpoint

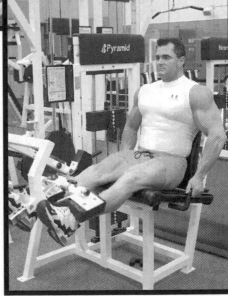

Quadriceps

Leg Machine Extensions

Starting Position:

- Sit on the leg press machine and tuck the front of your under ankles the pad

- Grasp the handles on the sides of the machine

Movement:

- Slowly raise the weight until your legs are straight and flex your quadricep muscles

- Slowly lower the dumbbells back to the starting position; repeat for the desired number of repetitions

Hamstrings

Barbell Straight-leg Dead Lifts

Start/Finish

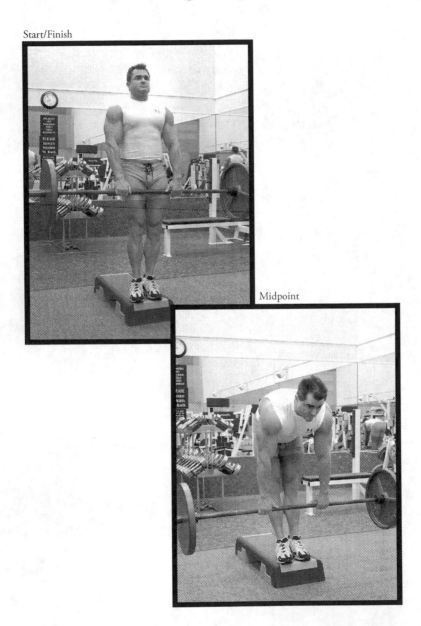

Midpoint

Hamstrings

Barbell Straight-leg Dead Lifts

Starting Position:

- Grasp the barbell with both hands approximately shoulder-width apart and your palms facing toward your body

- Stand up straight with your feet together while holding the barbell

Movement:

- Bend forward at your hips while keeping your head up and back straight and slowly lower the weight toward your ankles

- Slowly straighten your hips and raise the weight back to the starting position and flex your hamstring and gluteus muscles; repeat for the desired number of repetitions

Hamstrings

Leg Machine Curls

Start/Finish

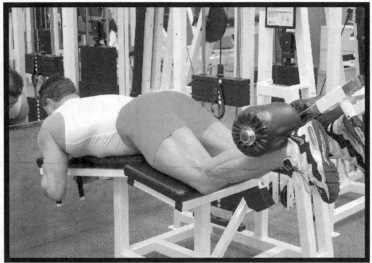

Midpoint

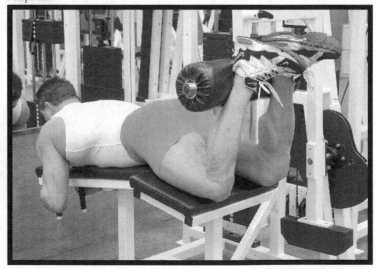

Hamstrings

Leg Machine Curls

Starting Position:

- Lie face down on the leg curl bench and tuck the backs of your ankles under the pads

Movement:

- Slowly raise the weight upward as far as you can and flex your hamstring muscles

- Slowly lower the weight back to the starting position; repeat for the desired number of repetitions

Hamstrings

Dumbbell Lunges

Start/Finish

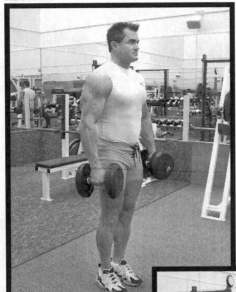

Midpoint

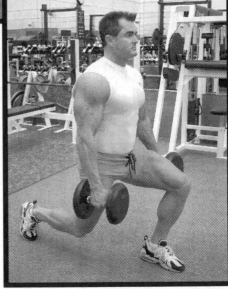

Hamstrings

Dumbbell Lunges

Starting Position:

- Grasp one dumbbell with each hand and stand in a upright position with your feet together

- Make sure you keep your head and chest up during the entire movement

Movement:

- Step forward with your left leg while bending your right knee until the upper part of your left leg is approximately parallel to the floor (your right knee should also be slightly bent and almost touch the floor, depending on how far forward you step)

- Using your left leg, raise your body weight back to the starting position

- After you have completed your desired number of repetitions, repeat the same movement with your right side

Calves

Seated Machine Calf Raises

Start/Finish

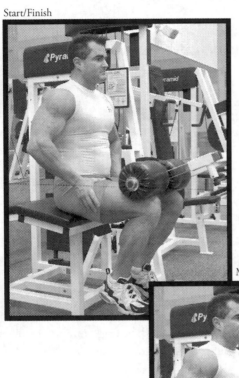

Midpoint

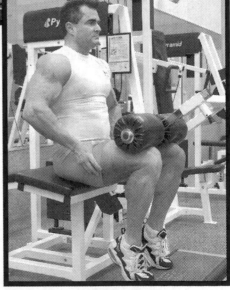

Calves

Seated Machine Calf Raises

Starting Position:

- Sit on seated calf machine, place the balls of your feet on the platform approximately six inches apart, and tuck your knees under the pads

Movement:

- Raise your heels upward as high as you can, lifting the weight toward the ceiling and flex your calf muscles

- Slowly lower the weight back to the starting position; repeat for the desired number of repetitions

Calves

Barbell Standing Calf Raises

Start/Finish

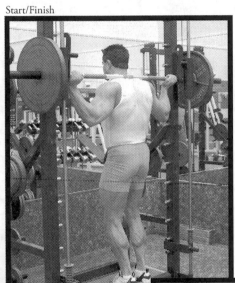

Midpoint

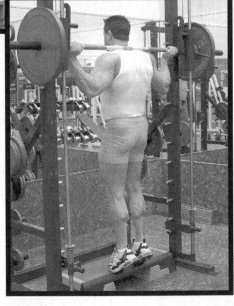

Calves

Barbell Standing Calf Raises

Starting Position:

- Place the barbell behind your neck on your shoulders (trap muscles)

- Grip the bar slightly wider than shoulder-width apart with your palms facing forward

- Position the balls of your feet on the platform approximately six inches apart

Movement:

- Raise your heels upward as high as you can, lifting the weight toward the ceiling and flex your calf muscles

- Slowly lower the weight back to the starting position; repeat for the desired number of repetitions

Calves

Dumbbell Standing Calf Raises

Start/Finish

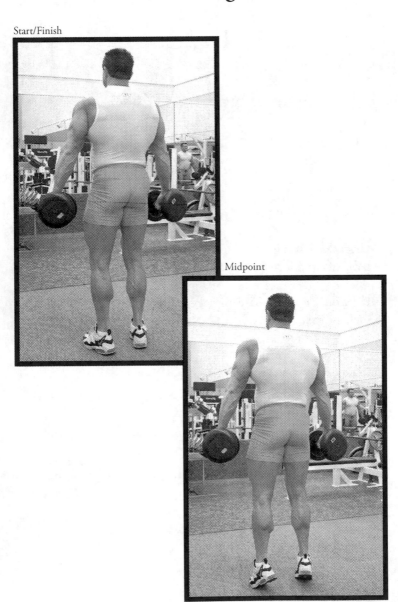

Midpoint

Calves

Dumbbell Standing Calf Raises

Starting Position:

- Grasp one dumbbell in each hand and stand up straight with your feet approximately six inches to shoulder-width apart

Movement:

- Raise up on your toes as high as you can and flex your calf muscles

- Slowly lower back to the starting position; repeat for the desired number of repetitions

9

Cardiovascular Exercise
(*Aerobic Conditioning*)

Aerobic means with air or oxygen. Aerobic conditioning involves exercising a large muscle group for a long duration at a low level of intensity. Aerobic exercise can help with weight loss and fat loss by increasing the amount of calories burned. For example, vigorous walking burns approximately 4 calories per minute; therefore, one hour of fast walking can burn as much as 240 calories. Running can burn approximately 6 to 8 calories per minute and burn as much as 240 calories in a half hour. Cardiovascular exercise helps condition the heart, helping to prevent heart disease, one of the top five causes of death nationally.

Benefits of Cardiovascular Exercise

- Contributes to the health of your heart muscle and blood vessels

- Increases the efficiency of your lungs and pumps more oxygen through your body

- Increases circulations throughout your entire body

- Increases metabolism

- Burns calories (reduces body fat)

- Improves the quality of muscle tone

- Help improve sleep

Examples of Cardiovascular Exercise

- Brisk Walking

- Jogging

- Cycling

- Swimming

- Aerobics classes

- Dancing

- Tennis

- Racquetball

- Roller-skating

- Hiking

Calculating Your Heart Rate

To calculate your heart rate yourself, you will need to count your heartbeats by taking your pulse. One way to take your pulse is to count for 15 seconds and than multiply that number by four; this will tell you how many times your heart beats in a one minute. To count your pulse yourself, use one of the following four locations.

1. **Neck**—Place your index finger and middle finger gently on the side of your neck near your throat (carotid artery).

2. **Wrist**—Place your first two fingers lightly on your wrist (radial artery) directly in line with the thumb.

3. **Temple**—Place your first two fingers on your temple just in front of your upper ear.

4. **Chest**—Place your palm over the left side of your chest.

If you do not want to take your own pulse, some cardiovascular machines have electronic pulse counters built into them. You can also purchase an inexpensive portable heart-rate monitor to carry with you.

Target Heart Rate

To receive the optimal benefit from your cardiovascular workout, you should be exercising within 50 to 75 percent of your maximum heart rate or "target heart rate" (THR). This zone is considered a moderate level of aerobic exercise. The level of your target heart rate is determined by your age, and will become lower the older you are. Average "resting heart rate" (RHR) is approximately 40 to 100 beats per minute, depending on your age and your health. Ideally, resting heart rate should be approximately 60 to 90 beats per minute, depending on your age and your health. Normal average resting heart rate for men is approximately 70 beats per minute, and for women is approximately 75 beats per minute.

The following chart illustrates estimated target heart rates based on various age groups. Find the age closest to yours, then read your target heart-rate zone.

Target Heart Rate Chart

Age	Target Heart Rate Zone: 50 to 75 percent	Average Maximum Heart: Rate 100 percent
20	100 to 150 beats per minute	200 beats per minute
25	98 to 146 beats per minute	195 beats per minute
30	95 to 142 beats per minute	190 beats per minute
35	93 to 138 beats per minute	185 beats per minute
40	90 to 135 beats per minute	180 beats per minute
45	88 to 131 beats per minute	175 beats per minute
50	85 to 127 beats per minute	170 beats per minute
55	83 to 123 beats per minute	165 beats per minute
60	80 to 120 beats per minute	160 beats per minute
65	78 to 116 beats per minute	155 beats per minute
70	75 to 113 beats per minute	150 beats per minute

You can also calculate your "maximum heart rate" (MHR) by subtracting your age from 220. For example, 220 minus 30 years of age equals 190 beats per minute MHR. This figure is within approximately 10 beats of your true target heart rate.

When you are beginning your cardiovascular exercise program, you should shoot for the lowest part of your target heart rate (50 percent) and gradually increase your level of intensity until you reach your higher target heart rate (75 percent).

If you do not want to take your pulse and use the target heart rate chart, you can rely on your instinct. If you can walk and talk at the same time and not be out of breath, you are probably not in your target heart-rate zone. However if you are breathing heavily and began to perspire, you can conclude that you have reached a sufficient level of intensity. If you are getting out of breath too quickly and have to keep slowing down or stopping or you feel lightheaded or dizzy, you are probably exercising too hard.

To receive a minimum benefit from cardiovascular exercise, the duration of your workout should last at least twenty minutes per session, three times a week, while exercising within your target heart-rate zone. When you continue aerobic conditioning for more than fifteen minutes, you begin to use fat as fuel much more efficiently. Aerobic conditioning is an excellent way to increase your metabolism, help control your weight and body fat, and strengthen your heart and lungs—as opposed to weight training, which for the most part is generally considered anaerobic exercise.

When constructing your exercise program, if you decide to do both cardiovascular exercise and weight training in the same workout session, in most situations I recommend that you do weight training exercise before you do cardiovascular exercise. Cardiovascular exercise uses stored carbohydrates in your body in the form of glycogen. Your body will burn the glycogen as fuel during cardiovascular exercise. If you do cardiovascular exercise prior to weight-training exercise, your muscles may have little or no glycogen left to fuel your weight training and your weight-training session will be less efficient. In addition, if you do your weight-training exercise prior to cardiovascular, exercise your body will burn some glycogen during weight training and this will give you a better opportunity to burn stored fat in your body for energy during your cardiovascular exercise.

10

Workout Schedules and Routines

Your workouts can be constructed in many different ways depending on how much time you are willing to devote. The following is a partial list of possible options.

Examples of Weekly Workout Schedules

#1—Three-Day, Beginner Workout Schedule- Train the entire body over a period of three separate days (Monday, Wednesday, Friday)

#2—Four-Day, Intermediate Workout Schedule- Train the entire body over a period of four separate days (Monday, Tuesday, Thursday, Friday)

#3—Five-Day, Advanced Workout Schedule- Train the entire body over a period of five separate days (Monday, Tuesday, Wednesday, Friday, Saturday)

Sample Weekly Workout Routines

Beginner Three-Day Routine: Workout #1

Three-Day Beginner Workout Schedule—Train the entire body over a period of three separate days (Monday, Wednesday, Friday)

Day One

Warm-up

- Straight Bar Stretch
- Hanging Bar Stretch
- Achilles Stretch
- Lunge Stretch

Chest

- Barbell Flat Bench Chest Press (2 sets for 10 reps)
- Chest Machine Flyes (2 sets for 10 reps)

Biceps

- Barbell Standing Bicep Curls (2 sets for 10 reps)
- Dumbbell Seated Bicep Curls (2 sets for 10 reps)

Triceps

- Cable Machine Tricep Push-downs (2 sets for 10 reps)
- Dumbbell Tricep Extensions (2 sets for 10 reps)

Cardiovascular

- Choose one of the following: treadmill, stair stepper, stationary bike, elliptical machine, rowing machine, aerobics class (thirty minutes or more, moderate pace)

Day Two

Warm-up

- Straight Bar Stretch
- Hanging Bar Stretch
- Achilles Stretch
- Lunge Stretch

Quadriceps

- Barbell Leg Squats (2 sets for 10 reps)
- Leg Machine Extensions (2 sets for 10 reps)

Hamstrings

- Barbell Straight-leg Dead Lifts (2 sets for 10 reps)
- Lying Machine Leg Curls (2 sets for 10 reps)

Calves

- Barbell Standing Calf Raises (2 sets for 10 reps)
- Seated Machine Calf Raises (2 sets for 10 reps)

Cardiovascular

- Choose one of the following: treadmill, stair stepper, stationary bike, elliptical machine, rowing machine, aerobics class (thirty minutes or more, moderate pace)

Day Three

Warm-up

- Straight Bar Stretch
- Hanging Bar Stretch
- Achilles Stretch
- Lunge Stretch

Back

- Seated Wide-grip Straight-bar Cable Pull-downs (2 sets for 10 reps)
- Seated V-grip Cable Rows (2 sets for 10 reps)

Shoulders

- Dumbbell Seated Shoulder Press (2 sets for 10 reps)
- Dumbbell Seated Side Lateral Raises (2 sets for 10 reps)

Abdominals

- Crunches (3 sets for 20 reps)
- Seated Bent-knee Leg Raises (3 sets for 10 reps)

Cardiovascular

- Choose one of the following: treadmill, stair stepper, stationary bike, elliptical machine, rowing machine, aerobics class (thirty minutes or more, moderate pace)

Intermediate Four-Day Routine: Workout #2

Four-Day Intermediate Workout Schedule—Train entire body over a period of four separate days (Monday, Tuesday, Thursday, Friday)

Day One

Warm-up

- Straight Bar Stretch
- Hanging Bar Stretch
- Achilles Stretch
- Lunge Stretch

Chest

- Barbell Flat Bench Chest Press (3 sets for 10 reps)
- Chest Machine Flyes (3 sets for 10 reps)

Biceps

- Barbell Standing Bicep Curls (3 sets for 10 reps)
- Dumbbell Seated Bicep Curls (3 sets for 10 reps)

Cardiovascular

- Choose one of the following: treadmill, stair stepper, stationary bike, elliptical machine, rowing machine, aerobics class (thirty minutes or more, moderate pace)

Day Two

Warm-up

- Straight Bar Stretch
- Hanging Bar Stretch
- Achilles Stretch
- Lunge Stretch

Quadriceps

- Barbell Leg Squats (3 sets for 10 reps)
- Leg Machine Extensions (3 sets for 10 reps)

Hamstrings

- Barbell Straight-leg Dead Lifts (3 sets for 10 reps)
- Lying Machine Leg Curls (3 sets for 10 reps)

Cardiovascular

- Choose one of the following: treadmill, stair stepper, stationary bike, elliptical machine, rowing machine, aerobics class (thirty minutes or more, moderate pace)

Day Three

Warm-up

- Straight Bar Stretch
- Hanging Bar Stretch
- Achilles Stretch
- Lunge Stretch

Back

- Seated Wide-grip Straight-bar Cable Pull-downs (3 sets for 10 reps)
- Seated V-grip Cable Rows (3 sets for 10 reps)

Shoulders

- Dumbbell Seated Shoulder Press (3 sets for 10 reps)
- Dumbbell Seated Side Lateral Raises (3 sets for 10 reps)

Cardiovascular

- Choose one of the following: treadmill, stair stepper, stationary bike, elliptical machine, rowing machine, aerobics class (thirty minutes or more, moderate pace)

Day Four

Warm-up

- Straight Bar Stretch
- Hanging Bar Stretch
- Achilles Stretch
- Lunge Stretch

Triceps

- Cable Machine Tricep Push-downs (3 sets for 10 reps)
- Dumbbell Tricep Extensions (3 sets for 10 reps)

Calves

- Barbell Standing Calf Raises (3 sets for 10 reps)
- Seated Machine Calf Raises (3 sets for 10 reps)

Abdominals

- Crunches (3 sets for 20 reps)
- Seated Bent-knee Leg Raises (3 sets for 10)

Cardiovascular

- Choose one of the following: treadmill, stair stepper, stationary bike, elliptical machine, rowing machine, aerobics class (thirty minutes or more, moderate pace)

Advanced Five-Day Routine: Workout #3

Five-Day Advanced Workout Schedule—Train entire body over a period of five separate days (Monday, Tuesday, Wednesday, Friday, Saturday)

Day One

Warm-up

- Straight Bar Stretch
- Hanging Bar Stretch
- Achilles Stretch
- Lunge Stretch

Chest

- Barbell Flat Bench Chest Press (4 sets for 10 reps)
- Dumbbell Incline Chest Press (4 sets for 10 reps)
- Chest Machine Flyes (4 sets for 10 reps)

Abdominals

- Crunches (3 sets for 20 reps)
- Decline Sit-ups (3 sets for 20 reps)
- Seated Bent-knee Leg Raises (3 sets for 10 reps)

Cardiovascular

- Choose one of the following: treadmill, stair stepper, stationary bike, elliptical machine, rowing machine, aerobics class (thirty minutes or more, moderate pace)

Day Two

Warm-up

- Straight Bar Stretch
- Hanging Bar Stretch
- Achilles Stretch
- Lunge Stretch

Quadriceps

- Barbell Leg Squats (4 sets for 10 reps)
- Leg Machine Press (4 sets for 10 reps)
- Leg Machine Extensions (4 sets for 10 reps)

Hamstrings

- Barbell Straight-leg Dead Lifts (4 sets for 10 reps)
- Lying Machine Leg Curls (4 sets for 10 reps)
- Dumbbell Lunges (4 sets for 10 reps per leg)

Cardiovascular

- Optional

Day Three

Warm-up

- Straight Bar Stretch
- Hanging Bar Stretch
- Achilles Stretch
- Lunge Stretch

Back

- Seated Wide-grip Straight-bar Cable Pull-downs (4 sets for 10 reps)
- Seated V-grip Rows (4 sets for 10 reps)
- Dumbbell One-arm Rows (4 sets for 10 reps)

Cardiovascular

- Choose one of the following: treadmill, stair stepper, stationary bike, elliptical machine, rowing machine, aerobics class (thirty minutes or more, moderate pace)

Day Four

Warm-up

- Straight Bar Stretch
- Hanging Bar Stretch
- Achilles Stretch
- Lunge Stretch

Shoulders

- Dumbbell Seated Shoulder Press (4 sets for 10 reps)
- Dumbbell Seated Side Lateral Raises (4 sets for 10 reps)
- Dumbbell Bent-over Lateral Raises (4 sets for 10 reps)

Calves

- Barbell Standing Calf Raises (4 sets for 10 reps)
- Seated Machine Calf Raises (4 sets for 10 reps)
- Dumbbell Standing Calf Raises (4 sets for 10 reps)

Cardiovascular

- Optional

Day Five

Warm up

- Straight Bar Stretch
- Hanging Bar Stretch
- Achilles Stretch
- Lunge Stretch

Biceps

- Barbell Standing Bicep Curls (4 sets for 10 reps)
- Dumbbell Seated Bicep Curls (4 sets for 10 reps)
- Cable Machine Bicep Curls (4 sets for 10 reps)

Triceps

- Lying Barbell Tricep Extensions (4 sets for 10 reps)
- Cable Machine Tricep Pushdowns (4 sets for 10 reps)
- Dumbbell Tricep Extensions – (4 sets for 10 reps)

Cardiovascular

- Choose one of the following: treadmill, stair stepper, stationary bike, elliptical machine, rowing machine, aerobics class (thirty minutes or more, moderate pace)

On the next page is a blank workout chart. You may want to make some extra copies to help you plan your daily workout schedule.

Workout Chart

Date	Exercise	Weight	Repetitions	Sets

The author at the Jan Tana Classic Bodybuilding Competition

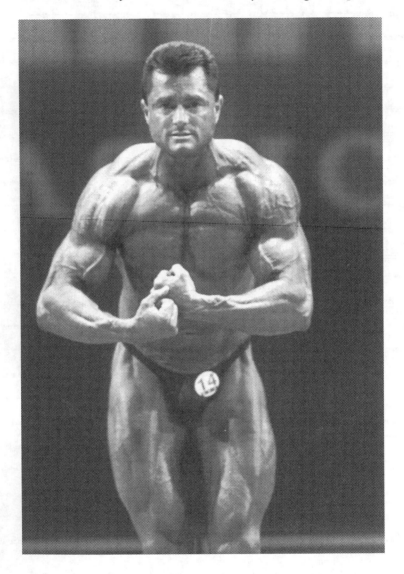

Photo by John Nafpliotis

11

Personalized Workout Profiles

Here are three different workout profiles. Each individual constructed a specific exercise program based on his or her own particular needs.

Personalized Workout Profile #1

Jim had worked in the corporate world since he graduated college: six days a week, ten to twelve hours a day. He was now sixty-two years old and had just retired. Suddenly the unexpected happened—Jim had a heart attack. Luckily, he survived, but he needed triple bypass surgery to clear the clogged arteries in his heart. The doctors told him that his sedentary desk job and his habit of eating rich foods had contributed to his extra weight and clogged arteries. Jim's physician recommended that he start an exercise program and clean up his diet to help avoid further health problems.

Jim's primary goal was to strengthen his heart muscle and keep his arteries clean. He also wanted to lose a little weight and tone up his muscles. He asked for my help.

First we decided to limit his restaurant dining and instead have him prepare healthier meals at home. Next we created a mild, three-day-a-week exercise program made up of approximately 70 percent cardiovascular and 30 percent weight training. We also agreed that, over time, he would progressively increase the intensity of his workouts.

Jim's Workout Program

Three-Day Workout Schedule (Monday, Wednesday, Friday)

Day One

Warm-up

- Straight Bar Stretch
- Hanging Bar Stretch
- Achilles Stretch
- Lunge Stretch

Chest

- Barbell Flat Bench Chest Press (3 sets for 10 reps)

Biceps

- Dumbbell Seated Bicep Curls (3 sets for 10 reps)

Triceps

- Cable Machine Tricep Push-downs (3 sets for 10 reps)

Cardiovascular

- Choose one of the following: treadmill, stair stepper, stationary bike, elliptical machine, rowing machine, aerobics class (thirty minutes or more, moderate pace)

Day Two

Warm-up
- Achilles Stretch
- Lunge Stretch

Quadriceps

- Leg Machine Extensions (3 sets for 10 reps)

Hamstring
- Lying Machine Leg Curls (3 sets for 10 reps)

Calves
- Seated Machine Calf Raises (3 sets for 10 reps)

Cardiovascular

- Choose one of the following: treadmill, stair stepper, stationary bike, elliptical machine, rowing machine, aerobics class (thirty minutes or more, moderate pace)

Day Three

Warm-up
- Straight Bar Stretch
- Hanging Bar Stretch
- Achilles Stretch
- Lunge Stretch

Back
- Seated Wide-grip Straight-bar Cable Pull-downs (3 sets for 10 reps)

Shoulders

- Dumbbell Seated Shoulder Press (3 sets for 10 reps)

Abdominals

- Crunches (3 sets for 15 reps)

Cardiovascular

- Choose one of the following: treadmill, stair stepper, stationary bike, elliptical machine, rowing machine, aerobics class (thirty minutes or more, moderate pace)

Personalized Workout Profile #2

Mary was thirty-five years old, married, and had three children. She had married when she was twenty years old and had devoted her life to caring for her family for the past fourteen years. Her daily diet was good but her three pregnancies had taken a toll on her body; she had gone from a firm one hundred sixteen pounds to one hundred forty-seven pounds.

All of Mary's children attended school during the day, which allowed time to exercise. Though her overall goal was to lose body fat and tone her muscles, Mary's primary target area was to tone and reshape her legs. She decided to join a local health club that was ten minutes from her house, where several of her friends were currently working out.

Mary's Workout Program

Four-Day Workout Schedule (Monday, Tuesday, Thursday, Friday)

Day One

Warm-up

- Achilles Stretch
- Lunge Stretch

Quadriceps

- Barbell Leg Squats (2 sets for 12 reps)
- Leg Machine Press (2 sets for 12 reps)
- Leg Machine Extensions (2 sets for 12 reps)

Hamstrings

- Barbell Straight-leg Dead Lifts (2 sets for 12 reps)
- Lying Machine Leg Curls (2 sets for 12 reps)
- Dumbbell lunges (2 sets for 12 reps)

Calves

- Barbell Standing Calf Raises (2 sets for 12 reps)
- Seated Machine Calf Raises (2 sets for 12 reps)

Cardiovascular

- Choose one of the following: treadmill, stair stepper, stationary bike, elliptical machine, rowing machine, aerobics class (forty minutes or more, moderate pace)

Day Two

Warm-up

- Straight Bar Stretch
- Hanging Bar Stretch
- Achilles Stretch
- Lunge Stretch

Chest

- Barbell Flat Bench Chest Press (2 sets for 10 reps)
- Chest Machine Flyes (2 sets for 10 reps)

Biceps

- Barbell Standing Bicep Curls (2 sets for 10 reps)
- Dumbbell Seated Bicep Curls (2 sets for 10 reps)

Triceps

- Cable Machine Tricep Push-downs (2 sets for 10 reps)
- Dumbbell Tricep Extensions (2 sets for 10 reps)

Cardiovascular

- Choose one of the following: treadmill, stair stepper, stationary bike, elliptical machine, rowing machine, aerobics class (forty minutes or more, moderate pace)

Day Three

Warm-up

- Straight Bar Stretch
- Hanging Bar Stretch
- Achilles Stretch
- Lunge Stretch

Back

- Seated Wide-grip Straight-bar Cable Pull-downs (2-sets for 10 reps)
- Seated V-grip Rows (2 sets for 10 reps)

Shoulders

- Dumbbell Seated Shoulder Press (2 sets for 10 reps)
- Dumbbell Side Lateral Raises (2 sets for 10 reps)

Abdominals

- Crunches (3 sets for 20 reps)
- Seated Bent-knee Leg Raises (3 sets for 10 reps)

Cardiovascular

- Choose one of the following: treadmill, stair stepper, stationary bike, elliptical machine, rowing machine, aerobics class (forty minutes or more, moderate pace)

Day Four

Warm up

- Achilles Stretch
- Lunge Stretch

Quadriceps

- Leg Machine Press (2 sets for 12 reps)
- Leg Machine Extensions (2 sets for 12 reps)

Hamstrings

- Lying Machine Leg Curls (2 sets for 12 reps)
- Dumbbell Lunges (2 sets for 12 reps)

Calves

- Barbell Standing Calf Raises (2 sets for 12 reps)
- Seated Machine Calf Raises (2 sets for 12 reps)

Cardiovascular

- Choose one of the following: treadmill, stair stepper, stationary bike, elliptical machine, rowing machine, aerobics class (forty minutes or more, moderate pace)

Personalized Workout Profile #3

For Bill, being overweight was all he had ever known. As far back as he could remember he had always been obese. His weight problem had negatively affected his life in many ways. His social life was nonexistent; in fact, Bill had never even been out on a single date. He often felt tired and sick. His doctor had recently told him that he needed to lose weight or he would probably encounter more severe health problems in the future.

"I am on a mission," were Bill's exact words to me. He eagerly volunteered to devote five days a week to his workout program. His primary goal was to lose a large amount of weight (body fat). The first adjustment we made was a total reconstruction of his diet. Bill was used to fast foods, binge eating, and "feel good" junk foods. We eliminated all foods that contained large amounts of fat, salt, and sugar.

As for his workout program, we decided to devote 80 percent to cardiovascular exercise and 20 percent to weight training. This allowed Bill to put a lot of emphasis on the aerobic conditioning that would help him shed excess weight. As he lost weight, we slowly adjusted the percentages of his workout to include more muscular conditioning (for toning) and less aerobic conditioning. I also suggested that it would be a good idea to take a set of before-and-after pictures, so he could look at the before pictures any time he felt the urge to binge on junk food.

Bill's Workout Program

Five-Day Workout Schedule
(Monday, Tuesday, Wednesday, Friday, Saturday)

Day One

Warm-up

- Straight Bar Stretch
- Hanging Bar Stretch
- Achilles Stretch
- Lunge Stretch

Chest

- Barbell Flat Bench Chest Press (2 sets for 12 reps)

Back

- Seated Wide-grip Straight-bar Cable Pull-downs (2 sets for 12-reps)

Cardiovascular

- Choose one of the following: treadmill, stair stepper, stationary bike, elliptical machine, rowing machine, aerobics class (forty minutes or more, light to moderate pace)

Day Two

Warm-up

- Straight Bar Stretch
- Hanging Bar Stretch
- Achilles Stretch
- Lunge Stretch

Quadriceps

- Leg Machine Extensions (2 sets for 12 reps)

Hamstrings

- Lying Machine Leg Curls (2 sets for 12 reps)

Calves

- Seated Machine Calf Raises (2 sets for 12 reps)

Cardiovascular

- Choose one of the following: treadmill, stair stepper, stationary bike, elliptical machine, rowing machine, aerobics class (forty minutes or more, light to moderate pace)

Day Three

Warm up

- Achilles Stretch
- Lunge Stretch

Cardiovascular

- Choose one of the following: treadmill, stair stepper, stationary bike, elliptical machine, rowing machine, aerobics class (sixty minutes or more, light to moderate pace)

Day Four

Warm-up

- Straight Bar Stretch
- Hanging Bar Stretch
- Achilles Stretch
- Lunge Stretch

Biceps

- Barbell Standing Bicep Curls (3 sets for 12 reps)

Triceps

- Cable Tricep Push-downs (2 sets for 12 reps)

Cardiovascular

- Choose one of the following: treadmill, stair stepper, stationary bike, elliptical machine, rowing machine, aerobics class (forty minutes or more moderate pace)

Day Five

Warm-up

- Achilles Stretch
- Lunge Stretch

Shoulders

- Dumbbell Seated Shoulder Press (2 sets for 12 reps)

Abdominals

- Crunches (2 sets for 12-reps)

Cardiovascular

- Choose one of the following: treadmill, stair stepper, stationary bike, elliptical machine, rowing machine, aerobics class (forty minutes or more, moderate pace)

The author at the Jan Tana Classic Bodybuilding Competition

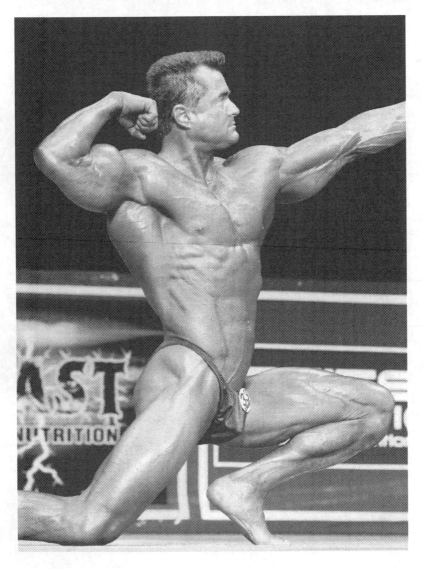

Photo by John Nafpliotis

12

Recuperation

Several factors can help speed your recuperation time between workouts and enhance the progress of your exercise program. The most obvious methods include rest, getting a sufficient amount of sleep, and following a high-quality, nutrition-packed diet. The following are optional methods to accelerate your recuperation process: stretching, ice, whirlpool, steam bath, sauna, and massage therapy.

Benefits of Stretching for Recuperation

(Refer to chapter 6 for stretching instructions and illustrations)

- Stimulates fresh blood and oxygen to joints and muscles that have overexerted

- Increases flexibility and range of motion (ROM)

- Helps reduce postworkout soreness

- Reduces stress

- Enhances mood

- Improves sleep

Benefits of Ice for Recuperation

Normally, if you have a strained or sprained a joint or muscle, it will become inflamed. As a result of the inflammation, an overabundance of blood is drawn to that location. The basic idea behind heat, stretching, massage, or ice is to move fresh blood and oxygen to the area to promote the healing process. Heat will dilate the blood vessels and draw more blood to the area, however might inflame it even more. The beauty of ice is that it constricts the blood vessels and reduces the inflammation. When your body resumes its regular temperature, the vessels resume back to normal and fresh blood moves in to help promote the healing process without increasing inflammation.

Ice is one of the best anti-inflammatory remedies used today. There are no side effects and it costs very little. Regular ice cubes placed into a plastic bag are generally too cold and end up leaking. Instead, you can purchase a "cold/hot gel pack" at any drug store. The gel pack is reusable, inexpensive, in addition it will conform to the shape of the body part you apply it to—I keep three of them in my freezer at home. You should apply ice for approximately twenty minutes a session several times a day.

Benefits of Whirlpools/Steam Baths/Saunas for Recuperation

These options all involve heat; approximately twenty minutes of heat per session is generally sufficient.

- Stimulates fresh blood and oxygen to joints and muscles that have overexerted

- Increases flexibility and range of motion (ROM)

- Helps reduce postworkout soreness

- Reduces stress

- Enhances mood

- Improves sleep

Benefits of Massage Therapy for Recuperation

Massage promotes a therapeutic response in our skin, muscles, connective tissues, ligaments, and tendons. Massage increases circulation and nourishes the body with fresh blood and oxygen. Blood is a healing tool of the body. The primary purpose of red blood cells is to carry oxygen from the lungs to all parts of the body, while white blood cells are part of the body's immune defense system. Increasing blood circulation helps promotes the healing process.

Massage helps eliminate waste products our bodies, products you may have acquired from poor diet, alcohol, environmental pollution, illness, et cetera. The lymphatic system is responsible for transporting our body's waste products and eventually disposes of them. Massage increases lymphatic circulation and speeds up the waste disposal process.

During exercise, muscles and nerve receptors become overfatigued and tissues become inflamed; ultimately, this creates delayed-onset muscle soreness. This usually occurs within twenty-four to seventy-two hours. The symptoms are fatigued, tight, sore, cramping muscles. Massage helps nourish these tissues with fresh blood and oxygen and can help speed up your recuperation time between workouts. The following is a list of health benefits that can be gained from receiving massage:

- Stimulates fresh blood and oxygen to joints and muscles that have overexerted

- Increases flexibility and range of motion (ROM)

- Helps reduce post workout soreness

- Reduces stress

- Enhances mood

- Improves sleep

- Enhances mood

- Reduces stress

- Increases energy

- Prevents injuries

- Improves flexibility

- Improves posture

- Improves alertness

- Improves muscle tone

- Improves skin tone

- Reduces lower back pain

- Flushes toxins

- Increases immunity

- Enhances nervous system

Overtraining Syndrome

I have been a victim of overtraining (over exercising) on several occasions. It is easy to do, especially if you become impatient and attempt to achieve your desired goals too quickly. Overtraining is considered counterproductive for several reasons. It may cause you to become overly fatigued. It can also be a major factor in promoting injuries. In addition it is possible to overtrain muscles to the point where they are unable to heal in a timely manner and will stop responding to exercise. Overtraining can also compromise your immune system and you may become sick. So remember, overtraining will only hinder your progress and set you on a downward spiral. Symptoms of overtraining may vary from one individual to the next. The following are some indications that your body may be the victim of overtraining:

- Chronic tiredness

- Irritability

- Lack of motivation

- Lack of recuperation (muscles always sore)

- Injuries (muscle cramps, tendentious, bursitis, sprains, strains)

- Difficulty sleeping, and difficulty rising in the morning

- Becoming sick often

- Irregular menstrual cycles (change in hormone levels)

Injury Care

If an injury occurs while exercising, such as a knee or ankle sprain or a strain, stop any physical activity as soon as possible and perform the following procedure called **RICE: R**est, **I**ce, **C**ompression, and **E**levation.

- **Rest**—Rest immediately and stop exercising to protect the injured or sore area from further injury.

- **Ice**—Ice the injured or sore area to reduce swelling, approximately twenty minutes per session.

- **Compression**—Compress the injured or sore area by wrapping it with an elastic bandage (such as an Ace bandage).

- **Elevation**—Elevate the injured or sore area with a pillow while applying ice to help reduce swelling.

If the injured or sore area does not feel better after a day or two, you may want to consult your physician or heath care provider for an evaluation. Above all else, listen to your body. It will let you know when there is a problem. If you feel overtrained, do not waste your time working out hard in a state of denial. Allow yourself to take some time off, or readjust your workouts.

The author at the Jan Tana Classic Bodybuilding Competition

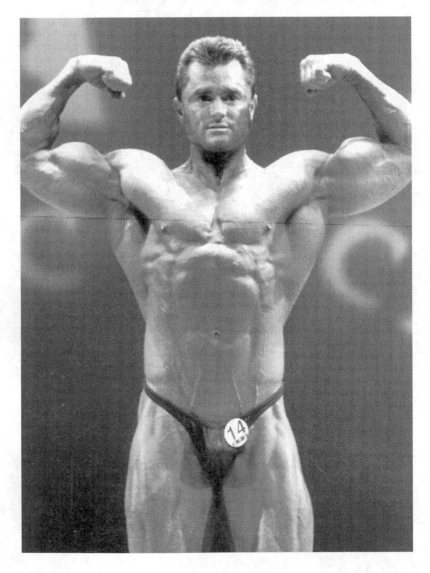

Photo by John Nafpliotis

13

Diet and Nutritional Guidelines

It is a good idea to consult your physician or heath care provider prior to starting a dietary program. Refer to the section in chapter 5 called Consulting your Physician for a list of possible reasons you may want to consult your physician prior to changing your diet.

Quality of Daily Diet

A proper diet and nutritional program will play a very important role in how quickly you progress with your exercise program and create positive changes in your physique. Try to avoid foods that contain large amounts of fat (saturated and trans fats), salt/sodium, and sugar: foods such as fast foods (cheeseburgers, fried foods, french fries) and junk foods (candy, pastries, potato chips, etc). Most of us already know which foods are good for us and which are not. For example:

- Plain toast versus toast with butter

- Plain tuna versus tuna with mayonnaise

- Egg white versus whole egg

- White meat versus red meat

- Broiled fish versus fried fish

If you use your common sense and do not lie to yourself, you will have won half the battle.

Nutrients

Nutrients are elements or compounds that are necessary for growth and other functions of the body. There are six essential nutrients needed to support the human body: proteins, carbohydrates, fats, minerals, vitamins, and water. Nutrients are generally divided into two categories: macronutrients and micronutrients.

Macronutrients include carbohydrates, proteins, fats, some minerals, and water. Macronutrients are needed daily in large quantities.

Micronutrients include vitamins and trace minerals; they are also needed daily, but in small quantities.

Essential nutrients are substances that must be obtained from our diets; the body cannot produce them on its own. Essential nutrients include vitamins, dietary minerals, essential fatty acids, and essential amino acids.

Nonessential nutrients are substances that do not have to be obtained from our diets. The body can produce these on its own.

Digestion and Absorption

Digestion and absorption are the processes in which food is broken down into small particles or molecules and absorbed into the body as nutrients. There are several stages involved in this process, both chemical and mechanical. Each phase of digestion transforms food into a slightly different form until it is ready for absorption. The following is a brief description of the different steps involved in both digestion and absorption.

1. The mouth and teeth chew the food into smaller particles.

2. The food is propelled through the digestive system.

3. Several different digestive enzymes are secreted and released.

4. Absorption takes place after the large, complex particles/molecules are transformed into smaller particles/molecules.

5. The small particles/molecules are absorbed into the blood stream and carried to the body's cells.

6. After nutrients and water are removed for use, undigested food and wastes are compacted and eliminated from the body.

Calories

A calorie is a measure of the energy content of foods. The energy that foods supply can be used immediately or stored for later use. When an individual consumes more than the number of calories the body needs at a given time, the excess calories will stored, mostly as fat—the result is weight gain. A pound of body fat is equal to 3,500 calories; therefore, ingesting an extra 200 calories a day for nine days may result in gaining approximately a half pound as fat.

It is nearly impossible to establish a specific, across-the-board policy for individuals concerning daily calorie intake. A specific calculation of calories added or cut to gain or lose weight is also difficult to predict. Many factors will determine your optimum daily calorie intake: age, gender, weight, genetics, metabolism, and physical activity. Energy requirements may vary from 1,000 to over 4,000 calories per day. Because calorie intake varies from person to person, the ranges for daily calorie intake listed below are only recommendations to use as a starting point.

Note: Eating an insufficient number of calories per day, less than your body requires, can cause your metabolism to slow down in order to adapt to the lower calorie intake. Because of your body is being deprived of calories, it tends to hold on to calories and store them as fat.

Average Daily Calorie Intake

Adult male: 2,000 to 3,000

Adult female: 1,800 to 2,400

Children:
(Ages 1 to 3) 1,300 to 1,600
(Ages 4 to 6) 1,600 to 1,800
(Ages 7 to 10) 2,000 to 2,200
(Ages 11 to 14) 2,200 to 2,500
(Ages 15 to18) 2,500 to 3,000

Personally, I do not count the amount of calories I take in daily; I prefer to rely on my instinct.

RDAs and DRIs

The previous Recommended Daily Allowances (RDAs) and the newer revised Daily Reference Intake (DRIs) are sets of guidelines illustrating the nutritional needs of normal, healthy people living in the United States and Canada. You can use these as general points of reference; these standards are not very specific regarding age, gender, weight, genetics, metabolism, and physical activity.

Carbohydrates, Proteins, and Fats

Your diet should primarily be made up of a combination of carbohydrates, proteins, and fats. The body uses these substances for growth, maintenance, repair, and energy. Specific amounts needed in a daily diet will vary by individual. Determining precise quantities for your own particular needs will depend on factors such as, age, gender, weight, genetics, metabolism, and physical activity. Exercising regularly will demand a higher level of performance from your body; therefore, you will need to give your body a better quality of fuel (carbohydrates, proteins, and fats).

Carbohydrates

Carbohydrates are made up of sugars. These sugars are metabolized in the body and converted into glucose, and are used as the main source of energy for the body.

There are two types of carbohydrates: complex carbohydrates (potatoes, rice, pasta, etc.) and simple carbohydrates (candy, pastries, fruits, etc.). Here are some guidelines for carbohydrates (or "carbs" for short).

- Approximately 40 to 60 percent of your daily diet should come from carbohydrates

- Approximately 75 percent of your carbohydrates should be complex carbohydrates

- Carbohydrates = 4 calories per gram

Sources of Carbohydrates

Complex Carbohydrates

Complex carbohydrates are often referred to as "starchy" foods. They are made up of multiple sugars bonded together in large molecules. Complex carbohydrates take longer to break down during the digestion and absorption process than simple carbs do. The slower absorption provides a long, steady supply energy for the body, as well as limiting the amount of sugar that is converted into fat and stored. As a result, there is less weight gain than with simple carbohydrates. In addition, complex carbohydrates usually contain more fiber, vitamins, and minerals than simple carbohydrates. The following is a partial list of foods that contain sources of quality complex carbohydrates. When available, read product labels for specific amounts of grams of complex carbohydrates included per serving.

- **Potatoes (white/red/sweet/yams):** 1 medium = approximately 25 grams of carbohydrates

- **Rice (brown/white):** 1/2 cup = approximately 35 grams of carbohydrates

- **Whole-grain breads/Cereals/Oatmeal:** 2oz = approximately 35 to 40 grams of carbohydrates

- **Pasta:** 2oz = approximately 40 grams of carbohydrates

Simple Carbohydrates

Simple carbohydrates are smaller molecules and are digested and absorbed faster than complex carbohydrates. Simple carbohydrates provide a quick, short burst of energy for the body and are likelier to be converted into fat. Natural simple carbohydrates such as fruits contain fiber, vitamins, and minerals. On the other hand, simple carbohydrates like refined sugars provide calories but lack fiber, vitamins, and minerals; they are considered "empty" calories and may promote more weight gain. Below is a partial list of foods that contain simple carbohydrates. When available, read product labels for specific amounts of grams of simple carbohydrates included per serving.

Simple Carbohydrates (Natural)

Fruit (fresh)

- **Apple:** approximately 18 grams of carbohydrates

- **Orange:** approximately 16 grams

- **Banana:** approximately 26 grams

- **Pear:** approximately 25 grams

Simple Carbohydrates (Refined Sugars)

- **Table sugar:** 1tbsp = approximately 11 grams of carbohydrates

- **Candy:** 1oz = approximately 20 to 25 grams

- **Cakes:** 1 piece = approximately 35 to 50 grams

- **Jam, Jellies, Preserves:** 1tbsp = approximately 14 grams

Protein

Protein is composed of twenty amino acids that are primarily responsible for maintenance and repair of many tissues in the body. Nine of the amino acids are called essential amino acids. Because the body does not make essential amino acids, they must come from the diet. Complete proteins containing all the essential amino acids are found in foods such as poultry, fish, and eggs.

The current RDA for protein is 0.8 grams per kilogram of body weight. An individual weighing 150 pounds would need approximately 55 grams of protein daily; however, some research suggests that you may need more protein when you increase your physical activity. Physically active individuals or those who desire to their increase muscle mass (endurance, strength, and power athletes) may need a higher amount of protein daily. These individuals may want increase that amount up to 1 gram or more of protein per pound of body weight daily, depending upon the intensity of their physical activity.

The average person can only absorb approximately 25 grams of protein at one time; however, age, gender, weight, genetics, metabolism, and physical activity can increase or decrease these numbers. Any unabsorbed protein is broken down and burned or stored as fat; therefore, protein intake should be separated by two to three hours. Guidelines for protein are:

- Approximately 20 to 30 percent of your daily diet should come from protein

- Protein = 4 calories per gram

Sources of Protein

The following is a partial list of foods that contain sources of good quality complete proteins. When available, read product labels for specific numbers of grams of protein included per serving.

Poultry 3oz = approximately 20 to 25 grams of protein

Fish: 3oz = approximately 20 to 25 grams

Egg whites: 1 large egg white = approximately 4 grams

Fat

Fats are complex molecules composed of fatty acids and glycerol. The body cannot manufacture some fatty acids; these are called essential fatty acids and must be consumed in your diet. There are several types of fats: saturated fats, trans fats, and unsaturated fats (these can be broken into polyunsaturated and monounsaturated fats). Below are guidelines for fats.

- Approximately 20 to 30 percent or less of your daily diet should come from fat

- Approximately 10 percent of your total calories from fat should come from polyunsaturated fats and approximately 10 to 20 percent of your total calories from fat should come from monounsaturated fats

- Approximately 7 to 10 percent of total calories from fat should come from saturated fats and trans fats

- Fat = 9 calories per gram

Sources of Fat

Listed below are descriptions of different types of fats and some examples of foods that contain them. When available, read product labels for specific types, amounts, and total grams of fats included per serving.

Saturated fats

Saturated fats ("bad fats") are typically found in animal fats, dairy, and some oils. They are usually solid at room temperature and contribute to elevating (LDL) "bad cholesterol" levels. High levels of LDL cholesterol in the blood can increase risk of heart disease, heart attack, and stroke. Following are some foods containing saturated fats.

- **Beef:** 3oz = approximately 1.5 to 10 grams of saturated fat

- **Pork:** 3oz = approximately 1.5 to 3 grams

- **Chicken (white meat):** 3oz = approximately 1 to 2 grams

- **Whole milk:** 1 cup = approximately 4.5 to 5 grams

- **Butter:** 1 tbsp = approximately 6 to 12 grams

- **Cheese (natural):** 1 oz = approximately 4 to 6 grams

- **Ice cream:** 1 cup = approximately 14 to 24 grams

Trans fats

Trans fats ("bad fats") are vegetable oils combined with hydrogen, creating a manmade fat. Trans fats can also elevate LDL levels. The following is a partial list of foods that contain trans fats. When available, read product labels for specific amounts of grams of trans fats included per serving.

- **Margarine:** 1 tbsp = approximately 0 to 8 grams of trans fats

- **French fries:** 3 oz = approximately 1 to 5 grams

- **Potatoes chips:** 2 oz = approximately 0 to 3 grams

- **Doughnuts:** 1 = approximately 3 to 5 grams

- **Cake (iced):** 1 slice = approximately 3 to 5 grams

Note: Saturated fats and trans fats are the main dietary factors that elevate LDL levels.

Unsaturated fats

Unsaturated fats ("good fats") contain essential fatty acids. Since your body cannot make essential fatty acids, you must obtain them through your diet. They help increase muscle, decrease body fat, promote cardiovascular health, and improve hormone levels—and much more. There are two types of unsaturated fats: polyunsaturated fats and monounsaturated fats. Polyunsaturated fats are not as good for you as monounsaturated fats; however, they are much better for you than saturated fats and trans fats. Some research has shown that consuming unsaturated fats in moderation may reduce your LDL blood cholesterol levels. The following is a partial list of foods that contain polyunsaturated and monounsaturated fats. When available, read product labels for specific amounts of grams of polyunsaturated and monounsaturated fats included per serving.

Polyunsaturated fats

Polyunsaturated fats are usually liquid both at room temperature and in the refrigerator. Polyunsaturated fats typically come from cold-water oily fish and plant sources.

Polyunsaturated fats can be divided into two categories: omega-3 and omega-6 fatty acids. Here are some sources of each:

Omega-3 fatty acids

Oily fish

- **Salmon:** 3.5 oz = approximately 0.1 to 1.4 grams of omega-3 fatty acids

- **Herring:** 3.5 oz = approximately 1.0 to 1.4 grams

- **Mackerel:** 3.5 oz = approximately 1.8 grams

- **Sardines:** 3.5 oz = approximately 1.4 grams

Omega-6 fatty acids

- **Corn oil:** 1 tbsp = approximately 7 grams of omega-6 fatty acids

- **Safflower oil:** 1 tbsp = approximately 8 grams

- **Sunflower oil:** 1 tbsp = approximately 8 grams

- **Flaxseed oil:** 1-tbsp = approximately 2 grams

Monounsaturated fats

Monounsaturated fats are usually liquid at room temperature; however, they may start to solidify in the refrigerator. Monounsaturated fats typically come from plant sources. Here are some of them:

- **Olive oil:** 1 tbsp = approximately 10 grams of monounsaturated fat

- **Canola oil:** 1 tbsp = approximately 8 grams

- **Peanut oil:** 1 tbsp = approximately 6 grams

- **Sesame oil:** 1tbsp = approximately 5 grams

Although polyunsaturated and monounsaturated fats have few adverse effects on LDL cholesterol levels, they should still be consumed in moderation. Eating large amounts of any fats adds extra calories. It is primarily calories from fat that cause people to be overweight, not calories from carbohydrates and protein. Remember, fat equals 9 calories per gram compared to carbohydrates and protein, which both equal 4 calories per gram.

In comparison, a note about alcohol: alcohol = 7 calories per gram, also more than either carbohydrates or protein.

Cholesterol

Cholesterol is found in both food and blood. Consuming foods that are high in saturated fats, such as animal fats and dairy, increases your levels of LDL ("bad" cholesterol).

These are the two types of cholesterol found in the blood.

- Low Density Lipoproteins (LDL—"bad")

- High Density Lipoproteins (HDL—"good")

LDL cholesterol is a waxy fat-like substance found in the blood. High levels of it can build plaque that can clog your arteries, causing hardening of the arteries, or atherosclerosis. This prevents the flow of blood and oxygen to your heart. High levels of LDL cholesterol in the blood may put you at risk for heart disease, heart attack, or stroke.

Here are guidelines for LDL and HDL:

- Healthy LDL blood levels should be less than 100 mg/dl

- Healthy HDL cholesterol blood levels should be approximately 45 mg/dl for males and 60 mg/dl females

The following is a chart of ranges for total cholesterol blood levels.

Cholesterol Blood Levels

Total Cholesterol Blood Levels	Classification
Less than 200 mg/dl	Optimal
200 to 239 mg/dl	Borderline high
240 mg/dl and above	High

Daily intake of foods containing cholesterol should be kept under 300 mg.

Triglycerides

Triglycerides are found in food and are manufactured in the body as well—they are another type of fat found in blood. When present at normal levels, they are essential for good health. High levels of triglycerides, however, may increase your risk of heart disease. The following is a chart of ranges for triglyceride blood levels.

Triglyceride Blood Levels

Total Triglycerides Blood Levels	Classification
Less then 150 mg/dl	Optimal
150 to 199 mg/dl	Borderline high
200 to 499 mg/dl	High
500 mg/dl and above	Very high

Fiber

Fiber is another important part of the diet. Here are some guidelines and benefits.

- Daily fiber intake should be at least 20 to 35 grams, up to 2 to 4 servings per day

- Fiber aids in the normal functioning of the digestive tract

- Fiber helps pass food through the intestines faster and helps maintain regular bowel movements and help prevent constipation

- Fiber helps burn body fat

- Fiber lowers the absorption of fat

- Fiber reduces appetite by making you feel full

- Fiber lowers blood cholesterol levels

- Fiber improves blood sugar levels

- Fiber helps reduce risk of heart attack

- Fiber helps reduce risk of adult-onset diabetes

Sources of Fiber

Bran cereals: 1/2 cup = 3 to 15 grams of fiber

- **All bran**

- **Complete bran flakes**

- **Grapenuts**

- **Oatmeal**

Breads/crackers/muffins made of whole wheat, rye, oats, or corn: approximately 3 to 5 grams of fiber

Vegetables (fresh are low in calories and contain antioxidants): approximately 1 cup = 4 to 5 grams of fiber

- **Broccoli**

- **Carrots**

- **Green beans**

- **Peas**

Fruits (those with edible skins are highest in fiber): approximately 3 to 4 grams of fiber

- **Apples**

- **Oranges**

- **Bananas**

- **Pears**

Legumes: approximately 1/2 cup = 6 to 7 grams of fiber

- **Baked beans**

- **Kidney beans**

- **Split peas**

- **Lima beans**

When available, read product labels for specific amounts of grams of fiber included per serving.

Sodium

Sodium (sodium chloride) is a component of salt. One gram of sodium is equal to 2.5 grams of salt. Ingesting an excessive amount of sodium over a long period of time can lead to high blood pressure, also called hypertension. This puts additional strain on your heart, which can cause health problems such as heart attack and stroke. In addition, a diet high in sodium can cause fluid retention, creating an increase in body weight. Some foods contain higher amounts of sodium than others do. Processed foods, canned foods, fast foods, junk foods, and most restaurant foods generally contain high amounts of sodium. When possible, check labels on processed foods for sodium amounts, and follow this guideline:

- Daily intake of sodium should be less than 2.4 grams (2,400 milligrams) per day; 2,400 milligrams of sodium is equal to 6 grams of salt or about a teaspoon.

Sugar

Foods contain many different types of sugars; however, glucose is the main sugar present in foods and in our blood. It is also our body's main source of energy. A diet of foods containing high amounts of sugar, or simple carbohydrates, can lead to high blood sugar levels—high amounts of glucose in the blood. After we eat carbohydrates, our body breaks them down into sugars, which are absorbed into the blood steam and distributed to the body's cells for energy.

It is important that blood sugar remains within specific levels: not too high and not to low. If blood sugar levels are consistently too high (hyperglycemia), it can lead to long-term health problems linked to diabetes. Diabetes is a condition in which the body's ability to produce insulin (a hormone secreted from the pancreas) is impaired. As a result, the body cannot properly break down and remove the sugar (glucose) in foods we eat from the bloodstream. This inhibits the supply of energy for the body's cells. Diabetes can lead to serious health conditions and damage many parts of the body including the heart, eyes, kidneys, nerves, blood vessels, teeth, gums, feet, and legs—it can even be life threatening. To help prevent diabetes, it is essential to maintain a healthy diet and a consistent exercise program. Treatment for diabetes includes proper medication, proper nutrition, and regular exercise.

If blood sugar levels drop too low (hypoglycemia), you risk experiencing shakiness, nervousness, weakness, faintness, anxiety, lethargy, irritability, and impaired mental functioning.

Blood sugar levels are normally lowest before your first meal of the day and higher after meals. Normal blood sugar levels range from 60 mg/dl to 120 mg/dl. Daily intake of sugar should be less than approximately 12 teaspoons or 48 grams.

The following is a chart containing blood sugar level ranges.

Blood Sugar Levels

Blood Sugar Levels	Classification
Less than 100 mg/dl	Optimal
120 to 126 mg/dl	Pre-diabetes
126 and higher mg/dl	Diabetes

Water

The human body is composed of approximately 50 to 70 percent water weight. For an average daily water intake, it is essential drink approximately eight 8-ounce glasses or more spread throughout the day. Drinking a sufficient amount of water daily is very important for maintaining good health. The following are some of the benefits of drinking adequate amounts of water daily.

- Helps regulate appetite

- Helps aid in digestion

- Helps prevent constipation

- Helps control body temperature

- Helps reduce hunger cravings

- Aids in circulation

- Helps transport nutrients

- Aids in nutrient absorption

- Replenishes body fluids lost through perspiration

- Prevents dehydration

- Flushes waste from kidneys

- Flushes toxins from body cells

- Keeps passageways moist (nose, mouth)

- Keeps eyes moist

- Keeps joints flexible

- Hydrates skin

Many people believe that if you drink a lot of water, your body will retain fluids and look puffy, but the reverse is true. If you do not drink enough water your body will tend to store more of it because it has been deprived of it: you will retain more fluids. If you drink plenty of water every day, your body will excrete it regularly. Insufficient hydration also slows down your metabolism and leads to fat storage.

The quality of the water you drink is important as well. Tap water from the faucet can contain many undesirable substances such as fluoride, lead, chlorine, pesticides, and parasites. Installing a filtration system on your faucet is one way to improve the quality of your drinking water. Another option is to purchase bottled water. There are many types available on the market: natural spring water, distilled water, mineral water, et cetera. Do your research and decide what the best choice is for you.

Tip: Drinking cold water can help burn calories, since a small amount of energy is required to raise the cold water to body temperature. You could burn up to 50 to 150 calories a day by drinking a half gallon to a gallon of cold water throughout the day.

Summary of Recommended Daily Nutrient Intake

Carbohydrates

- Approximately 40 to 60 percent of your daily diet should come from carbohydrates

- Approximately 75 percent of your carbohydrates should come from complex carbohydrates

Protein

- Approximately 20 to 30 percent of your daily diet should come from good-quality complete proteins

Fat

- Approximately 20 to 30 percent or less of your daily diet should come from fat

- Approximately 10 percent of your total calories from fat should come from polyunsaturated fats and approximately 10 to 20 percent of your total calories from fat should come from monounsaturated fats

- Approximately 7 to 10 percent of total calories from fat should come from saturated fats and trans fats

Cholesterol

- Daily intake of foods containing cholesterol should be kept under 300 mg.

Fiber

- Daily fiber intake should be at least 20 to 35 grams, up to two to four servings per day

Sodium

- Daily intake sodium should be less than 2,400 mg per day, or about a teaspoon of salt.

Sugar

- Daily intake of sugar should be less than approximately 12 teaspoons (48 grams)

Water

- Daily intake of water should be approximately eight 8-ounce glasses, or more, spread throughout the day

The author and (Actress/Model) Carol Grow filming a TV commercial for MuscleTech

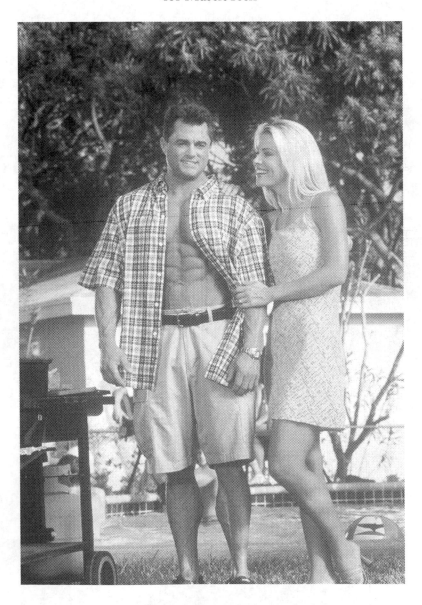

14

Diet Tips

Food Labels

Food manufactures are required by the Food and Drug Administration to include "Nutritional Facts" labels on almost all foods. These labels provide consumers with accurate information about food products and can help you plan a healthier, better-balanced diet to fit your own personal needs. The following page illustrates a sample Nutritional Facts label for whole-wheat pasta. Read it over, get familiar with the information it contains, and try to get in the habit of reviewing these labels for foods you purchase.

Whole Wheat Pasta

Nutrition Facts
Serving size 2oz (56g ¾ cup) dry
Servings per container about 7

Amount Per Serving

Calories 180 Calories from Fat 5

% Daily Values*

Total Fat 1g **1%**

 Saturated Fat 0g 0%

 Trans Fat 0g

Cholesterol 0mg **0%**

Sodium 0 mg **0%**

Total Carbohydrate 42g **14%**

 Dietary Fiber 6g **24%**

 Sugars 1g

Protein 6g

Iron 10% Thiamin 35%

Riboflavin 15% Niacin20%

Folate (Folic Acid) 30%

Not a significant source of vitamin A, vitamin C, and calcium

* Percent Daily Values are based on a 2,000 calorie diet. Your daily values

may be higher or lower depending on your calorie needs.

Calories 2,000 2.500

Total Fat Less than 65g 80g

Sat Fat Less than 20g 25g

Cholesterol Less than 300mg 300mg

Sodium Less than 2,400mg 2,400mg

Total Carbohydrate 300g 375g

Dietary Fiber 25g 30g

Calories per gram:

Fat 9 Carbohydrate 4 Protein 4

Reference Values for Nutrition Labeling

(Based on a 2000-calorie intake; for adults and children four or more years of age)

Nutrient	Unit of Measure	Daily Values
Total fat	grams (g)	65
Saturated fatty acids	grams (g)	20
Cholesterol	milligrams (mg)	300
Sodium	milligrams (mg)	2400
Potassium	milligrams (mg)	3500
Total carbohydrate	grams (g)	300
Fiber	grams (g)	25
Protein	grams (g)	50

Grocery List

In order to help make your diet a success, it is essential to create a specific and detailed grocery list prior to going food shopping. If you do not purchase any junk food, you will not have it in your house, and if you get a craving for junk food you will have none to eat. I personally like to buy large quantities of food at a time; this makes it easy to create all my healthy meals. In addition, I like to precook and prepackage my meals as much as possible. This allows for easy access and I can take my meals with me on the road.

Timing Your Meals

Breakfast

Make sure that you do not skip breakfast or your first meal after a long sleep. Your body has probably gone about eight to twelve hours without any nutrition. If you skip breakfast, you will probably have no energy for work, or for working out. In addition, your body might store the next meal you have because it has been deprived for too long between meals.

Eating Small, Frequent Meals

Eat at least four to six small meals per day, and eat approximately every two to three hours. Eating small, frequent meals can also help with weight loss and fat loss, by increasing the body's metabolism. After we eat, insulin (hormone) levels generally increase. With smaller meals, these levels do not increase as much as they would with larger meals, and this helps reduce fat accumulation. Listed below are some of the benefits of eating smaller meals more frequently.

- Helps increase your metabolism

- Helps suppress your appetite

- help utilize nutrients more efficiently

- Helps improve absorption of food

Eating Before Sleeping

Avoid large meals before bedtime. Your metabolism will slow before and during sleep, thus hindering your ability to burn calories efficiently. If your capability to burn calories becomes hindered, the opportunity to store fat will be increased.

Lowering Carbohydrate Intake

If your goal is to maintain your current body weight or body composition, you can balance your carbohydrates, protein, and fat, using the information provided in this chapter. If your goal is to structure your diet to lose weight or body fat, the obvious was is to decrease your daily calorie intake. However, you may want to make more specific adjustments, such as decreasing your daily carbohydrate intake.

Carbohydrates are the body's primary source of energy, so if you lower your carbohydrate intake it will allow your body to use excess body fat as fuel for your energy needs. This technique can help expedite your fat loss. For example, if you are consuming 30 or 40 grams of carbohydrates per meal, drop them in half to 15 or 20 per meal. You can do this for a couple of meals or a couple of days, and then return to normal intake for a couple of meals or days. Use your instinct to help determine how often you want to alternate your carbs from half to full portions. If at any time you begin to feel tired, sluggish, or lightheaded, you can bring your carbs back up to your normal intake.

Always try to keep your protein at your normal intake level; this will help prevent your body from using your muscles as fuel for your body's energy needs. Low carbs are the basic theme behind the popular Atkins Diet and South Beach Diet.

And remember, when trying to lose body weight or body fat, avoid foods containing large amounts of saturated fats, trans fats, sodium, and sugar.

Cheating

I recommend that you do not make your diet too strict to follow; you will probably become miserable and resentful. And don't make your guidelines too unrealistic by deciding, for example, that you will never eat junk food again as long as you live. You should allow yourself to occasionally cheat on some meals. Consider this example: If you were to eat four to six meals per day, seven days per week, this would total twenty-eight to forty-two meals per week. If you eat three or four "cheat meals" out of this number, the good meals will certainly outweigh the not-so-good. Cheating on a couple of meals a week will be a reward for your good diet efforts and will have a minimal negative impact on your physique. Life is too short to make set ridiculous guidelines.

You may wish to seek the advice of a nutritional specialist, such as a registered dietitian, depending on how serious you are about constructing a proper diet and nutritional program.

Summary of Basic Diet Guidelines

- Avoid foods that contain excessive amounts of, saturated fat, sodium, and sugar.

- Do not skip breakfast

- Avoid overeating at one sitting

- Eat smaller meals more frequently

- Avoid meals before bedtime

- Drink a sufficient amount of water

The author at Jan Tana Classic Bodybuilding Competition

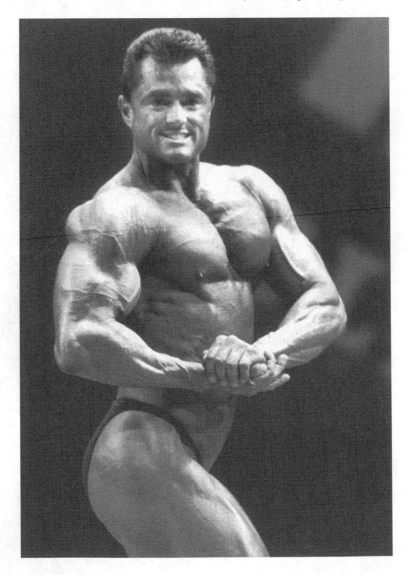

Photo by John Nafpliotis

15

Sample Daily Diets

Note: The specific amounts of carbohydrates, protein, and fats needed in a daily diet will vary by individual. Refer to previous chapters to help determine the precise quantities for your own particular needs.

Sample Daily Diet #1

(Four Meals Daily)

Meal 1

- Egg white omelet
- Oatmeal or whole-grain cereal
- Fresh fruit

Meal 2

- Broiled chicken
- Brown rice
- Mixed fresh vegetables or salad

Meal 3

- Broiled fish
- Baked potato
- Mixed fresh vegetables or salad

Meal 4

- Broiled turkey
- Whole-wheat rice cakes
- Fresh fruit

Note: A meal-replacement bar or shake can be substituted for a meal.

Sample Daily Diet #2

(Five Meals Daily)

Meal 1

- Egg white omelet
- Oatmeal or whole-grain cereal
- Fresh fruit

Meal 2

- Broiled chicken
- Brown rice
- Mixed fresh vegetables or salad

Meal 3

- Broiled fish
- Baked potato
- Mixed fresh vegetables or salad

Meal 4

- Broiled turkey
- Whole-wheat rice cakes
- Fresh fruit

Meal 5

- Broiled chicken
- Yams
- Mixed nuts

Note: A meal-replacement bar or shake can be substituted for a meal.

Sample Daily Diet #3

(Six Meals Daily)

Meal 1

- Egg white omelet
- Oatmeal or whole-grain cereal
- Fresh fruit

Meal 2

- Broiled chicken
- Brown rice
- Mixed fresh vegetables or salad

Meal 3

- Meal replacement bar or shake

Meal 4

- Broiled fish
- Baked potato
- Mixed fresh vegetables or salad

Meal 5

- Broiled turkey
- Whole-wheat rice cakes
- Fresh fruit

Meal 6

- Broiled fish
- Baked yams
- Mixed nuts

Note: A meal-replacement bar or shake can be substituted for a meal.

On the next page is a blank daily diet chart. You may want to make some extra copies to help you plan your daily meal schedule.

Daily Diet Chart

Meal 1	
Meal 2	
Meal 3	
Meal 4	
Meal 5	
Meal 6	

The author at the NPC National Bodybuilding Competition

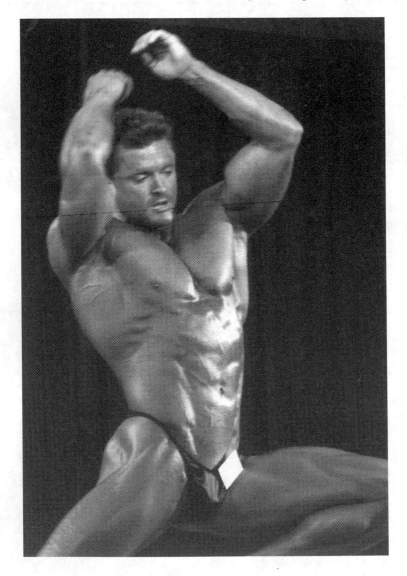

Photo by JM Manion (www.jmmanion.com)

16

Nutritional Supplements

It is a good idea to consult your physician or heath care provider prior to using any dietary supplements. Refer to the section in chapter 5 called Consulting Your Physician for a list of possible reasons you may want to consult your physician prior to starting your dietary supplement program.

What are nutritional supplements? Supplements are powders, pills, or tablets that contain nutrients. "Supplement" is the key word; they should be used in addition to a well-balanced diet to supplement what you may have missed in your food. Supplementation can help you maintain a healthy body. They can also help you with fat loss and muscle toning. Used in conjunction with your exercise program, supplements will assist you in enhancing your athletic performance and producing positive results in your physique.

Note: Dosages for individual supplements may vary depending on age, gender, body weight, metabolism, physical activity, and life style. Nutritional supplements are scientifically engineered. Therefore, you should follow the recommended dosages printed on the label and use as directed.

Vitamin and Mineral Supplements

Vitamins and minerals are essential nutrients for maintaining a healthy, functioning body. In today's society the methods involved in processing foods can destroy a portion of the original vitamin and mineral content. In addition, fast foods, cooked foods, and poorly constructed diets can contain insufficient amounts of the nutrients needed to maintain healthy. You can use vitamin and mineral supplements as insurance to replace what you may have missed in your daily diet.

At the same time that your diet may be lacking in nutrients, there are many factors that can deplete the vitamins and minerals you do ingest:

- Poor diet

- Overexercising

- Overworking

- Stress

- Illness

- Lack of sleep

- Pollution

- Alcohol and drugs

Vitamins

There are two types of vitamin supplements:

Fat-soluble: these require fats or oils for your body to absorb them.

Water-soluble: these require only water for absorption.

The following is a partial list of vitamin supplements with brief descriptions of their benefits. After reviewing the list, you may want to consider researching specific ones in greater depth and adding them to your daily diet according to your own personal needs.

Vitamin A is fat-soluble. It is needed for eye, teeth, and gum health and is a good antioxidant to protect against skin disorders.

Vitamin B-1 (thiamine) is water-soluble. It helps convert carbohydrates into energy.

Vitamin B-2 (riboflavin) is water-soluble and helps convert carbohydrates, proteins, and fats into energy.

Vitamin B-3 (niacin) is water-soluble. It aids in the proper function of the nervous digestive systems and helps the body produce energy.

Vitamin B-5 (pantothentic acid) is water-soluble and helps release energy from foods. It also strengthens the immune system.

Vitamin B-6 (pyridoxine) is water-soluble and helps support the cardio-vascular system. It also helps convert carbohydrates, proteins, and fats into energy and aids in building blood cells.

Vitamin B-9 (folic acid) is water-soluble and helps prevent birth defects, heart disease, and strokes.

Vitamin B-12 (cobalamin) is water-soluble and promotes production of red blood cells. It also helps convert carbohydrates and proteins into energy and benefits the nervous system.

Vitamin C is water-soluble. It assists the immune system and is also a good antioxidant. It helps heal tissues and promotes healthy teeth and gums.

Vitamin D is fat-soluble. It aids in the absorption of calcium, thereby helping to maintain strong bones and teeth.

Vitamin E is fat-soluble and aids in the circulation of red blood cells. It helps prevent heart disease and also acts as an antioxidant.

Vitamin K is fat-soluble. It is needed to maintain the proper clotting of blood. It also helps to maintain healthy bones and helps to prevent osteoporosis.

Vitamin Recommendations

Vitamins: Comparison of Current RDIs, New RDIs and URLs			
VITAMIN	*CURRENT RDI**	*NEW RDI***	*UL***
Vitamin A	5000 IU	900 mcg (3000 IU)	3000 mcg (10,000IU)
Vitamin C	60 mg	90 mg	2000 mg
Vitamin D	400 IU (10mcg)	15 mcg (600 IU)	50 mcg (2000 IU)
Vitamin E	30 IU (20 mg)	15 mg #	1000 mg
Vitamin K	80 mcg	120 mcg	ND
Thiamin	1.5 mg	1.2 mg	ND
Riboflavin	1.7 mg	1.3 mg	ND
Niacin	20 mg	16 mg	35 mg
Vitamin B-6	2 mg	1.7 mg	100 mg
Folate	400 mcg (0.4 mg)	400 mcg from food, 200 mcg synthetic ##	1000 mcg synthetic
Vitamin B-12	6 mcg	2.4 mcg ###	ND
Biotin	300 mcg	30 mcg	ND
Pantothenic acid	10 mg	5 mg	ND
Choline	Not e stablished	550 mg	3500 mg

* The Reference Daily Intake (RDI) is the value established by the Food and Drug Administration (FDA) for use in nutrition labeling. It was based initially on the highest 1968 Recommended Daily Allowance (RDA) for each nutrient, to assure that needs were met for all age groups.

** The Reference Daily Intake (RDI) are the most recent set of recommendations established by the Food and Nutrition Board of the Institute of Medicine, 1997–2001. They replace the previous RDAs, and may be the basis for eventually updating the RDIs. The value shown here is the highest DRI for each nutrient.

***The Upper Limit (UL) is the upper-level intake considered to be **safe** for use by adults, incorporating a safety factor. In some cases, lower ULs have been established for children.

Historically vitamin E conversion factors were amended in the DRI report, so that 15 mg is defined as the equivalent of 22 IU of natural vitamin E or 33 IU of synthetic vitamin E.

It is recommended that women of childbearing age obtain 400mcg of synthetic folic acid from fortified breakfast cereals or dietary supplements, in addition to folate.

It is recommended that people over 50 meet the B-12 recommendations through fortified foods or supplements, to improve bioavailability.

ND Upper limit not determined. No adverse effects observed from high intakes of nutrient.

Council for Responsible Nutrition (www.crnusa.org)

Minerals

Minerals are inorganic elements that are found in nature. They are needed to support a healthy body and must be acquired through our diet. There are two types of minerals: trace (small amounts) and major (large amounts). The following is a partial list of mineral supplements with brief descriptions of their benefits. After reviewing it, you may want to consider researching some of the minerals further and adding them to your daily diet according to your own personal needs.

Trace Minerals

Chromium helps breakdown glucose (simple sugars) in the body and converts glucose to energy.

Copper promotes the formation of bones, hemoglobin, and red blood cells. Copper also plays a role in the production of energy for cells and increases the body's energy level.

Iron is needed for the production of red blood cells and transporting oxygen. Iron helps prevent fatigue and helps promote body growth. Women lose more iron (through menstruation) than men, so need to take in more iron than men do.

Selenium helps vitamin E as an antioxidant and helps prevent premature aging. It also helps maintain the elasticity of tissues.

Zinc promotes wound healing, immune function, protein synthesis, glucose utilization, and insulin production.

Major Minerals

Calcium is an essential mineral needed to maintain healthy teeth and strong bones.

Magnesium plays a role in nerve and muscle function in addition to maintaining healthy teeth and strong bones.

Phosphorus is responsible for creating normal teeth and bones.

Potassium helps regulate the water balance within the body and cells.

I prefer to take a take a multi (several nutrients combined) and timed-release vitamin and mineral supplement. The timed-release aspect supplies the nutrients in intervals over an extended period of time, keeping doses in your system longer (two to six hours) for better absorption.

Mineral Recommendations

Minerals: Comparison of Current RDIs, New RDIs, and URLs			
MINERAL	*CURRENT RDI**	*NEW RDI***	*UL****
Calcium	1000 mg	1300 mg	2500 mg
Iron	18 mg	18 mg	45 mg
Phosphorus	1000 mg	1250 mg	4000 mg
Iodine	150 mcg	150 mcg	1100 mcg
Magnesium	400 mg	420 mg	4000 mg #
Zinc	15 mg	11 mg	40 mg
Selenium	70 mcg	55 mcg	400 mcg
Copper	2 mg	0.9 mg	10 mg
Magnesium	2 mg	2.3 mg	11 mg
Chromium	120 mcg	35 mcg	ND
Molybdenum	75 mcg	45 mcg	2000 mcg

* The Reference Daily Intake (RDI) is the value established by the Food and Drug Administration (FDA) for use in nutrition labeling. It was based initially on the highest 1968 Recommended Daily Allowance (RDA) for each nutrient, to assure that needs were met for all age groups.

** The Reference Daily Intake (RDI) are the most recent set of recommendations established by the Food and Nutrition Board of the Institute of Medicine, 1997–2001. They replace the previous RDAs, and may be the basis for eventually updating the RDIs. The value shown here is the highest DRI for each nutrient.

***The Upper Limit (UL) is the upper-level intake considered to be **safe** for use by adults, incorporating a safety factor. In some cases, lower ULs have been established for children.

Upper-limit magnesium applies only to intakes from dietary supplements or pharmaceutical products, not including intakes from food or water.

ND Upper limit not determined. No adverse effects observed from high intakes of nutrient.

Council for Responsible Nutrition (www.crnusa.org)

Herbs

Herbs have been around for many years and have been used as alternative natural healing methods. The following is a partial list of herbal supplements with brief descriptions of their benefits. After reviewing the list, you my want to consider adding some to your daily diet according to your own personal needs.

Aloe Vera can be used as a topical healing gel for burns or rashes; it can also be used to moisturize and maintain healthy skin.

Asian Ginseng helps provide energy and endurance, and helps fight fatigue.

Echinacea is said to enhance the body's immune system.

Ephedra (also called Ephedrine and Ma Huang) is a stimulant that has been used for weight control, as an energy boost, and to enhance athletic performance.

Garlic helps maintain proper healthy cardiovascular function.

Ginko Biloba helps supply increased blood flow and oxygen to the brain.

Green Tea can be used as a blood antioxidant and detoxifier.

Saw Palmetto helps men maintain a healthy prostate.

St. John's Wart helps maintain a positive mood in people who suffer from mild depression and anxiety.

Valerian helps provide relief for people who suffer from insomnia, anxiety, and stress.

High-Tech Supplements

- **Protein shakes and bars** increase muscle mass and repair.

- **Meal replacement shakes and bars** substitute for a regular meal.

- **Thermogentics** burn fat, increase energy, and boost metabolism.

- **Creatine** enhances muscle, strength, recovery, and body weight—men only.

- **Prohormones** are testosterone boosters that enhance muscle, strength, recovery, and body weight—men only.

- **L-glutamine** prevents muscle breakdown, aids in muscle recuperation.

- **Chondroitin** is anti-inflammatory and enhances joint repair.

- **Glucosamine** is anti-inflammatory and enhances joint repair.

At one time or another, I have utilized all the high-tech supplements mentioned above in conjunction with my diet and exercise program. I choose to cycle individual supplements at different times of the year, depending on what my specific goals are at that particular time. Here is a list of my personal favorites:

Meal Replacement shakes and bars are convenient when you are on the go and do not have time to eat properly. Regular meals are generally a better choice; however, most people's lifestyles are too busy to allow time to eat solid balanced meals. Meal replacement shakes and bars are an excellent alternative and most certainly better than skipping a meal altogether.

Thermogentics naturally boost your metabolism and also contain fat-burning ingredients for losing fat without sacrificing muscle. They can also help prevent excess carbohydrates from being converted into fat and reduce hunger cravings. One of my favorite qualities of thermogentics is that it creates a substantial increase in energy level, giving you an extra kick for your workouts, especially when you have had a tough day or are tired and feel like skipping a workout.

Proper supplementation will help give you that added edge when it comes to creating and maintaining a lean, toned body. Do your research and choose the supplements that will fit your own particular program. Be sure to select a reputable brand-named company. Remember, you only get what you pay for.

The Food and Drug Administration (FDA) regulates dietary supplements, vitamins, minerals, and herbs. The charts included in this chapter listing recommended dosages for vitamin and mineral supplements are provided by the Council for Responsible Nutrition. They compare the previous Recommended Daily Allowance (RDA) to the more recent Reference Daily Intake (RDI); in addition, the chart also includes the Upper Limit (UL). The ULs are recommendations for the highest level of daily nutrient intake that is not likely to cause any adverse health risks in a general healthy population. You can use these as a general point of reference. These standards are not very specific regarding age, gender, weight, genetics, metabolism, and physical activity. Nutritional supplements are scientifically engineered. You should follow the recommended dosages printed on the label and use as directed.

The author and John Wood, Jr. at a photo shoot for *MuscleMag*

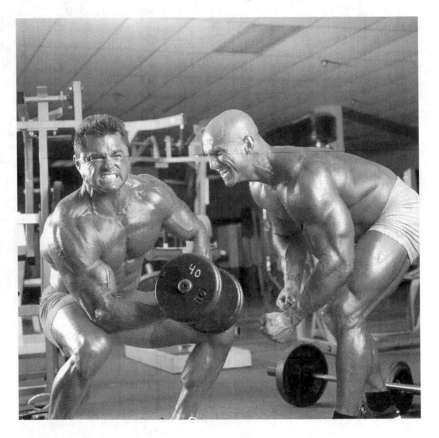

Photo by Ralph DeHaan (www.ralphdehaan.com)

17

Positive Thinking and Attitude

When I was competing in gymnastics, one of my coaches handed me some literature containing methods to achieve positive thinking and positive attitude. I have referenced them numerous times over the years, particularly when I was having difficulty making good decisions in many different types of situations. I share them here in hopes that you, too, will benefit from these methods.

Attitude

Attitude is more important than anything else. It is more important than the past, education, money, circumstances, failures, successes, and especially what other people think, say, or do. It is more important than appearance, giftedness, or skills. It will make or break a business ... a home ... a friendship ... an organization. The remarkable thing is you have a choice everyday of what your attitude will be. We cannot change our past ... we cannot change the actions of others. We cannot change the inevitable. The only thing we can change is our attitude. Life is 10 percent what happens to us and 90 percent how we react to it. To quote Thomas Edison, "Invention is 10 percent inspiration and 90 percent perspiration." Simply put, we are, each and every one of us the master of our own destiny.

Author Unknown

Mental Edge

Do you think like a winner or a loser?

It is no accident that certain people and certain teams have a way of winning more than others. In his best-selling book, *Winners and Losers*, Sydney Harris says that successful people in all walks of life—athletics, school, work, or play—seem to share a certain special way of thinking about things that set them apart from the rest of the pack. Harris basically says that winners see things differently than losers do, and that is why they win. How do you know if you think like a winner or a loser? Here is a little test adapted from his book that might surprise you.

A winner listens.
A loser just waits for his turn to talk.

A winner makes commitments.
A loser makes promises.

A winner works harder than a loser and has more time.
A loser is always "too busy" to do what is necessary.

A winner says, "Let's find out."
A loser says, "Nobody knows."

A winner says, "There ought to be a better way to do it."
A loser says, "That's the way it's always been done here."

A winner learns from his mistakes and tries something different.
A loser quits trying.

A winner hopes for a miracle after everything has failed.
A loser hopes for a miracle before anything has been tried.

A winner goes through a problem.
A loser goes around it and never gets past it.

A winner takes a big problem and separates it into smaller parts so that it can be more easily manipulated.

A loser takes a lot of little problems and rolls them together until they are unsolvable.

A winner knows how much he still has to learn, even when he is considered an expert by others.

A loser wants to be considered an expert by others before he has even learned enough to know how little he knows.

When **a winner** makes a mistake he says, "I was wrong."
When **a loser** makes a mistake he says, "It wasn't my fault."

A winner shows he's sorry by making up for it.
A loser says, "I'm sorry" but does the same thing next time.

A winner is sensitive to atmosphere around him.
A loser is sensitive only to his own feelings.

A winner forgives.
A loser is too petty to forgive.

A winner stops talking when he has made his point.
A loser goes on until he has blunted his point.

A winner seeks for the goodness in a bad man, and works with that part of him.

A loser looks for only the badness in a good man, and therefore finds it hard to work with anyone.

A winner knows that people are kind if you give them a chance.
A loser feels that people will be unkind if you give them a chance.

A winner acts the same toward those who can be helpful and those who can be of no help.

A loser fawns on the powerful and snubs the weak.

A winner tries never to hurt people, and does so rarely, when it serves a higher purpose.

A loser never wants to hurt people intentionally, but does so all the time, without even knowing it.

A winner knows when the price of winning comes to high.
A loser is over eager to win what he cannot handle or keep.

A winner knows what to fight for and what to compromise on.
A loser compromises on what he shouldn't and fights for what isn't worth fighting about.

A winner has a healthy appreciation for his abilities and a keen awareness of his current limitations.
A loser is oblivious to both his true abilities and his true limitations.

A winner would rather be admired than liked, although he would prefer both.
A loser would rather be liked than admired, and is even willing to pay the price of mild contempt for it.

A winner rebukes and forgives.
A loser is too timid to rebuke and too petty to forgive.

A winner in the end gives more than he takes.
A loser dies clinging to the illusion that winning means taking more than you give.

A loser becomes bitter when he's behind and careless when he is ahead.
A winner keeps his equilibrium no matter what position he happens to find himself in.

A loser believes in fate.
A winner believes that we make our fate by what we do or fail to do.

A loser leans on those stronger than himself, and takes him frustrations out on those weaker than himself.
A winner leans on himself, and does not feel imposed upon when he is leaned on.

A loser prides himself on his "independence" when he is merely being contrary, and prides himself on his "teamwork" when he is merely being a conformist.

A winner knows which decisions are worth an independent stand, and which should be gone along with.

A loser blames "politics" or "favoritism" for his failure.

A winner would rather blame himself than others, but he doesn't waste time on any kind of blame.

A loser thinks there are rules for winning and losing.

A winner knows that every rule in the book can be broken except for one: Be who you are and become who you were meant to be, which is the only winning game in the world.

More on Attitude

(Adapted from Earl Nightingale audio tape *The Magic Word*)

It is our attitude at the beginning of a task which, more than anything else, will affect its successful outcome.

It is our attitude toward life which will determine life's attitude toward us.

We are interdependent! It is impossible to succeed without others. And it is our attitude toward others that will determine their attitude toward us.

Before a person can achieve the kind of life he wants, he must become that kind of individual—he must think, act, talk, walk, and conduct himself in all of his affairs —as would the person he wishes to become.

The higher you go in any organization of value, the better the attitudes you will find.

Your mind can only control one thought at a time. Since there is nothing to be gained by holding on to negative thoughts, hold successful, positive thoughts.

The deepest craving of human beings is to be needed, to feel important, and to be appreciated. Give it to them, and they'll return it to you.

Part of a good attitude is to look for the best in new ideas—and look for the good ideas everywhere.

Don't waste your time broadcasting personal problems. It probably won't help you—and it cannot help others.

Don't talk about your health unless it's good—unless you are talking to your doctor.

Radiate an attitude of well-being, of confidence, of a person who knows where he going. You'll find good things start to happen right away.

Lastly, for the next thirty days, treat everyone with whom you come in contact as the most important person on earth. If you do this for thirty days, you'll do this for the rest of your life.

Publishing permission granted from Diana Nightingale. (www.earlnightingale.com)

18

Childhood Obesity

Within the last two decades, childhood obesity has reached epidemic proportions. Observe today's general youth population and you will see that the following statistics are very accurate. Obesity among children has risen by approximately 40 percent. Childhood obesity has increased 54 percent in children age six to eleven, and 39 percent in adolescents ages twelve to seventeen. One out of every five teenagers is said to be overweight. A child possessing an excessive accumulation of body fat is considered obese. If total body weight is more than 25 percent fat in boys and more than 32 percent fat in girls, they are considered obese.

If an individual has a weight problem as a child, that does not necessarily mean he or she will be heavy as an adult. However, the risk of being obese as an adult is increased as the child ages. Children reaching the state of obesity by the age of six increase their risk of being overweight as an adult by approximately 50 percent, while for obese adolescents the risk increases to an alarming of 70 to 80 percent.

Causes of Childhood Obesity

Childhood obesity can result from several factors, nutritional, psychological, and physiological. Most childhood obesity is due to calorie intake that exceeds energy output; only a small percentage of childhood obesity is associated with hormonal or genetic disorders. Lack of physical activity and poorly constructed diet are the major contributing factors for weight gain in children. Today's average child spends several hours a day watching television, playing video games, and sitting at computers—and junk foods will normally accompany these types of activities. Becoming overweight should come as no surprise to children who are consistently engaged in sedentary activities and who have poor eating habits.

Experts have found that infants who have overweight mothers are generally less active and become heavier than normal-weight infants with normal-weight mothers. Research also shows that a child's risk of becoming obese is increased when one or both parents are overweight. This is usually due to the eating and exercise habits modeled by the parent(s).

Problems with Childhood Obesity

Physical Health Disorders

Obesity has become a very serious health problem for children. The following is a list of health risks linked to childhood obesity.

- Increased risk of cardiovascular disease

- Increased risk of diabetes

- High blood pressure (hypertension)

- High cholesterol levels

- Orthopedic problems (increased stress on joints)

- Sleep disorders

- Skin disorders

- Low energy level

Negative Psychological Effects

The following is a list of some common psychological problems found to be associated with growing up as an obese child.

- Low self-esteem

- Low self-confidence

- Negative self-image

- Introverted personality (withdrawn from peers)

- Fear of failure

- Depression

- Negative impact on school grades, ultimately affecting college and career choices

- Lack of social life involving friends, dating, and ultimately marriage

In many cases, these negative psychological issues may be carried into adulthood and have an impact on the quality of career opportunities; they may also lead to fewer opportunities for romantic relationships and marriage. Statistically, due to lack of social development, children who are overweight upon entering adulthood are less likely to get a higher education or earn as much as people of normal weight.

Treatment

Preventing childhood obesity is easier than treating it. A child's eating and exercise habits are easier to correct at a young age and become harder to correct as an adult. As a parent, make sure you have sufficient knowledge concerning proper child nutrition, beginning with breast-feeding or bottle-feeding on through the introduction of solid foods. Parents should take the time to learn and practice proper nutrition and exercise habits themselves.

If your child is obese, he or she should be evaluated by a physician. Keep in mind that there are no safe dieting medications for children. Approach the treatment of obesity through behavioral modification by establishing a proper daily diet and increased daily physical activity. Positive reinforcement throughout every phase of these lifestyle changes will help in the overall success of your child's efforts.

You must set safe, realistic goals for weight loss for your overweight child. Try not to make your goals unattainable; this will discourage your child. If the goal is too high, the child may become overwhelmed or discouraged. Start with a goal of five or ten pounds, losing approximately one to five pounds a month depending on the age and weight of the child.

Establishing a Proper Diet for Your Child

Review the guidelines for proper diet and nutrition in chapter 13. You can use this as a model for establishing a basic diet for your child; however, make adjustments to food amounts based on age and weight.

Try not to alienate the child when enforcing a new diet. The entire family should become involved with healthy eating habits. Overfeeding is possible beginning in infancy, whether you are breast-feeding or bottle-feeding, but it has been proven more prevalent with bottle-feeding. After two years of age, you can safely replace whole milk for skim milk.

A good rule to remember is this: if you do not buy junk food and bring it home, it will not be available to eat. A child's diet should get approximately 30 percent of its calories from fat. Here is a list of suggestions to help prevent childhood obesity.

- Do not use food as a reward for good behavior

- Do not use food as a reward for finishing a regular meal

- Do not use food to comfort a child

- Do not allow a child to eat junk food between meals

- If a child is hungry between meals, offer them fruit instead of salty or sugary snacks

- Do not allow a child to access food without your permission

- Do not force a child to finish every meal or eat when they are not hungry

- Limit eating at fast-food restaurants

- If you create good eating habits early on, they could last a lifetime

---

Average Daily Calorie Intake for Children

Children (Ages)
(1 to 3) 1,300 to 1,600
(4 to 6) 1,600 to 1,800
(7 to 10) 2,000 to 2,200
(11 to 14) 2,200 to 2,500
(15 to 18) 2,500 to 3,000

Establishing Physical Activities for Your Child

Physical activity at a young age can become a good habit for life. A good exercise program or a variety of physical activities can help a child burn body fat, increase energy, and help maintain a healthy weight.

First, regulate the amount of time your child spends watching television, playing video games, and sitting at the computer. You will need to incorporate several types of physical activities into their schedules: for example, outdoor activities such as family walks, cycling, et cetera. Remember, it is best if the entire family becomes involved to help in setting good examples. The age of the child will help you choose the appropriate activities. For children under six years of age, many preschools or private gymnastic schools offer classes in "preschool phys-ed movement," starting as early as two years old. The primary focuses of these classes are as follows:

- Teach passive exercise movements

- Teach body awareness

- Improve coordination skills

- Increase flexibility

- Mousercise (aerobics classes for children, ages two and a half to five)

- Learn how to interact in an organized exercise classroom situation

The following is a short list of possible options for children six years of age and above (depending upon the maturity of the individual).

Individual Activities

- Playing ball

- Walking

- Jogging

- Cycling

- Roller-skating

- Swimming

Classroom Activities

- Dance classes

- Gymnastic classes

- Martial arts classes

- Aerobic classes

Organized Sports Activities

- Soccer

- Cheerleading

- Track and field

- Baseball

- Football

- Basketball

- Field hockey

- Ice hockey

- Tennis

Negative impacts resulting from childhood obesity, whether physiological or psychological, are certainly worth avoiding. Remember, preventing childhood obesity is easier than treating it!

Conclusion

You are in control of developing your own exercise and diet program. When constructing your program, try to choose weight training and cardiovascular exercises that are fun and interesting to you. Making your workouts more fun will help hold your interest and will not seem like a chore. Achieving good results from your workouts will be based on the high level of intensity and consistency you put into them. It is like putting money in the bank: the more you put in, the more you will have in the end.

Your entire workout should be progressive, built upon over time. Do not attempt to "build in a day." Trying to do too much too soon will be too difficult and will only discourage you. Consistency, not one big workout, equals success.

You are the pilot of your own ship; you will create your own destiny. Only you can choose to help yourself. You are the one in control of your lifestyle and only you can determine if you want to exercise and eat properly.

Remember, the exercise and diet program you develop will not only increase the quality of your physique; it will enhance your self-esteem, self-confidence, and energy level. Always maintain a positive attitude and believe in yourself, and there will be nothing you cannot accomplish.

Good luck and good health!

Notes

Notes

Notes

Bibliography

Books

Balch, James F MD and Phyllis A. Balch, CNC. *Prescription for Natural Healing.* New York: Avery Publishing Group, 1997

Corbin, Charles B., Gregory J. Welk, Ruth Lindsey, and William R. Corbin. *Concepts of Physical Fitness.* New York: McGraw-Hill, 2003

Levandoski, Richard, MD; Harold Tabai, DO; William Gomez, MD; Edward Silverman, DO; Bill Schull, MD; Amy Freedman, MD; Stanley Beloff, DPM; and Brian Halpern, MD. *Step Aerobics Personal Fitness Trainer & Nutritional Manual.* AAAI/ISMA, Inc.: Pennsylvania

Levandoski, Richard, MD; Harold Tabai, DO; William Gomez, MD; Edward Silverman, DO; Bill Schull, MD; Amy Freedman, MD; Stanley Beloff, DPM; and Brian Halpern, MD. *Studies in Exercise Science.* AAAI/ISMA, Inc.: Pennsylvania

Martini, Fredrick PhD. *Fundamentals of Anatomy and Physiology.* New Jersey: Prentice Hall, 1989

Miller-Keane. *Encyclopedia & Dictionary of Medicine, Nursing, & Allied Health.* Philadelphia: W.B. Saunders Company, 1997

Nichols, Frank. *Theory and Practice of Body Massage*. New York: Milady Publishing Corporation, 1987

Papalia, Diane E. and Sally Wendkos Olds. *Human Development*. New York: McGraw-Hill, 1981

Prudden, Bonnie. *Pain Erasure*. New York: Ballantine Books, 1980

Seeley, Rod R., PhD, Trent D. Stephens, PhD, and Phillip Tate, DA. *Anatomy & Physiology*. St. Louis: Mosby-Year Book, Inc., 1995

Whitney Noss, Eleanor and Eva May Nunnelley Hamilton. *Understanding Nutrition*. Minnesota: West Publishing Company, 1981

Web Sites

American Academy of Family Physicians, *Working for family medicine working for you*, <http://www.aafp.org/online/en/home.html> (6 April 2007).

American Heart Association, *Live and Learn*, <http://www.americanheart.org/presenter.jhtml?identifier=1200000> (19 September 2007).

Council for Responsible Nutrition, *The Science Behind the Supplements*, *<http://www.crnusa.org/index.html>* (14 June 2007).

Discovery Health, *Disease, Pregnancy, Fitness, Weight Loss*, <http://health.discovery.com/> (23 July 2007).

DrLam.com, *An insider's Guide to Natural Medicine*, <http://www.drlam.com/> (17 July 2007).

Healthlink, *Medical College of Wisconsin*, <http://www.healthlink.mcw.edu/> (9 April 2007).

Joanne Larson MS RD LD, *Ask the Dietitian*, <http://www.dietitian.com/index.html> (7 July 2007).

Life Clinic, *Health Management Systems*, <http://www.lifeclinic.com/default.asp>
(9 August 2007).

Medline Plus, *Health information from the National Library of Medicine*, 18 September 2007, <http://medlineplus.gov/> (19 September 2007).

National Dairy Council, *A leader in nutrition research and education since 1915,* <http://www.nationaldairycouncil.org/NationalDairyCouncil/> (14 August 2007).

Net Wellness, *Consumer Health Information,* <http://www.netwellness.org/> (3 September 2007).

Shape up America, *Healthy Weight for a Healthy Life,* <http://www.shapeup.org/prof/child.php> (25 April 2007).

U.S. Food and Drug Administration, *Center for food Safety & Applied Nutrition,* <http://www.cfsan.fda.gov/list.html> (8 September 2007).

U.S. Food and Drug Administration, *Consumer Health Information,* <http://www.fda.gov/default.htm> (12 June 2007).

WebMD, *Better Information. Better Health,* <http://www.webmd.com/> (18 June 2007).

Women's Health America, *The Natural Hormone Experts,* <http://www.womenshealth.com/home> (3 June